T0381129

EMOTIONAL INTELLIGENCE
FOR
PHYSICAL FITNESS

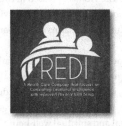

The REDI-Network
Tackles our American Obesity Crises

Jay Houston, Ph.D.

BALBOA.PRESS
A DIVISION OF HAY HOUSE

Balboa Press books may be ordered through booksellers or by contacting:

Balboa Press
A Division of Hay House
1663 Liberty Drive
Bloomington, IN 47403
www.balboapress.com
844-682-1282

Because of the dynamic nature of the Internet, any web addresses or links contained in this book may have changed since publication and may no longer be valid. The views expressed in this work are solely those of the author and do not necessarily reflect the views of the publisher, and the publisher hereby disclaims any responsibility for them.

The author of this book does not dispense medical advice or prescribe the use of any technique as a form of treatment for physical, emotional, or medical problems without the advice of a physician, either directly or indirectly. The intent of the author is only to offer information of a general nature to help you in your quest for emotional and spiritual well-being. In the event you use any of the information in this book for yourself, which is your constitutional right, the author and the publisher assume no responsibility for your actions.

Any people depicted in stock imagery provided by Getty Images are models, and such images are being used for illustrative purposes only. Certain stock imagery © Getty Images.

Print information available on the last page.

ISBN: 979-8-7652-5330-4 (sc)
ISBN: 979-8-7652-5329-8 (e)

Library of Congress Control Number: 2024912247

Balboa Press rev. date: 07/16/2024

ABOUT THE AUTHOR

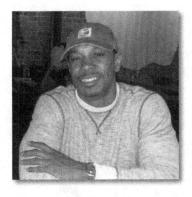

The swirling combination of
19 years of
Pharmaceutical & Biotech Sales,
7 years of
Academic & Biotech Research
in Molecular Biology
& Computational Chemistry,
9 years as a fitness instructor/trainer
As well as
A life-long curiosity of psychology has inspired
this author to create a new genre of books.
CEO and Founder of The REDI Network.

CONTENTS

SECTION 4: IMPACT HEALTH SYSTEMS

SECTION 1
Realize the source

CHAPTER 1

Why Write this book?

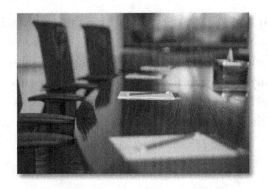

October 2019. Downtown Philadelphia.

A healthcare conference is being held inside of an upscale hotel for patients with a rare genetic lung disease.

That conference became the impetus for this book on the numerous emotional obstacles blocking collective fitness goals related to the obesity crisis in The United States.

How could a two-day meeting on a thoroughly unrelated topic lead to a book on psychological solutions for systemic American struggles with fitness and obesity? The answer begins with why we're in Philly in the first place.

My attendance was on behalf of my employer – one of the leading manufacturers of treatment for this genetic lung disorder. Also in attendance: Disease-state-expert researchers, physicians, and nurses.

All these health-care professionals were giving speeches and seminars throughout both days. There were patients from all over this country who not only learned from these experts, but also bonded with one another, united against the disease.

Amidst the formality of the Philadelphia conference, the true inspiration for this book occurred from conversations during breaks in hallways and at lunch tables.

I was simply curious. I was brand new to working within this disease state. So, I took the opportunity to speak directly with several patients during the scheduled breaks built into the conference schedule. I asked them casually *how many of their family members* had been tested for this rare disease? Because the test itself is extremely easy, reasonably rapid, and free of charge. It's a simple cheek swab at your local doctor's office.

My thoughts were:

> "This disease is genetic. It can become a very serious health threat if misdiagnosed. So surely, patients' families had all been tested, right?"

To my astonishment and alarm, most of the patients I spoke with said their own siblings and grown children not only had *not* been tested but *didn't want to* get tested.

Further than curious, I was becoming a bit distressed. This disease is not an insignificant matter at all. Why on earth would anyone *not* want to do a free and simple test when they know a close family member *has* the genes that can lead to this disease?

Perhaps you can presume why.

Realize the source: Because of the emotion: fear.

Not just fear of finding out whether they had inherited the genes for the disease (which is extremely unlikely, hence the designation of being a *rare* disease). But a fear that they may be required to alter their lifestyle: quit smoking, lose weight, adjust their diet, become less sedentary.

This is the same fear which makes some of us avoid our scale at home or postpone going to the doctor's office altogether. And make no mistake, as simple as this genetic test is, you still must schedule it at the doctor's office, which leads to trepidation as well.

Back to the conference. Here's what led to this book. At lunch, one sweet, elderly patient uttered a simple yet profoundly perfect response to my growing incredulousness. She said:

> "Honey, people don't want to change. They just want
> to put their feet up when they get home from work
> and watch their TV shows."

She was 100% spot on. But for me, my despondency (at the lack of people getting a free and easy cheek swab test) was intensified because of the incredible number of resources assembled at *this* conference, for *these* patients with *this* disease.

The depth and diversity of information at this event was immense:

- World-renowned genetic researchers.
- Tenured, hospital nurses who had been working decades in this disease state.
- A long-standing, highly respected non-profit organization dedicated solely to these patients nationwide.
- Multiple pharmaceutical companies sponsoring the occasion (including my employer) at booths stuffed with data on our products and empathy from highly trained and highly educated personnel.

All these entities were committed to giving advice and care. They were also scientifically arming patients with knowledge. Not to be forgotten, there was an emotional support network attending this event: other patients themselves. It was a sensational network of people.

And yet, *fear* of getting out of a comfort zone rendered this conference – bearing all the hallmarks of a supportive networking platform - under-attended by people who could benefit from all these numerous resources. It's not that the efforts of all the organizers were wasted, but so many *more* people could have been assisted.

The conference was only 2 days. With a whirlwind of information and people it went by rapidly. It was time to drive home. As I strolled out of the hotel and across the parking lot and climbed into my car, those conversations with the patients regarding their families weighed on my mind more than the subject matter itself.

And on this ensuing drive home to Washington, DC, the thoughts kept growing as to how the same scenario seen at this conference unfolds throughout our nation. Meaning: staggering resources met with thunderous apathy. It happens not just with rare genetic diseases but with so many people across the health and fitness spectrum.

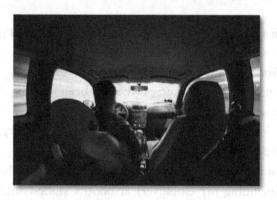

I kept my phone and my numerous music apps off. Just my thoughts and the highway. I started reflecting on my time as a personal trainer and a Pilates instructor. I thought about my own struggles to get into "elite" conditioning. I thought about how I've been trying (and failing) to help one of my dear friends to lose 100+ pounds.

Through the tolls and tunnels of interstate 95, over the bridges and bypasses, I recalled countless conversations I've had with health-care professionals through the years. Their struggles, their despair to beg patients to lose weight and not be dependent on medications always stood out to me in their uniformity of despair. Two decades of my employment within the field-based healthcare industry became an engine of rumination. It propelled towards the pseudo homonym: REDI.

The REDI Network creates a discussion
platform for delicate topics.

This book will illustrate how we can:
Realize the source.
Examine our subconscious.
Discuss self-awareness & self-regulation.
Impact the systems affecting
our outcomes.

This topic for this book:
Utilizing Emotional
Intelligence to increase
Fitness Goals

Thoughts careened towards our entire nation; our strong desires to "get in shape" are overruled by individual deeper, stronger desires to rectify what's in our subconscious.

And our subconscious *drives us*. It controls our focus far more than we realize. It can take us to destinations it *wants* to visit.

Nearing home, the thoughts had crystallized from that conference in Philadelphia. Akin to that conference, our subconscious' desires and decisions *render* the numerous amounts of *resources* available to help us with our health: under-utilized.

In stark contrast to that conference, it's not that we can't commence attempts to change our health, we can't manage to maintain our plans. We can't finish.

Again, step one: **R**ealize the source. So many of our individual inabilities to complete our journeys towards our fitness goals are because our conscious' desires do not always align with our subconscious' needs.

Emotional Intelligence (EQ) gives us the tools to increase our individual awareness of our subconscious' fears and irrational beliefs. EQ can raise the level of our own self-awareness and self-regulation.

EQ graces us with a safe space to discuss emotionally charged topics.

- Individually, are we completely in control of our decision making? How do conscious fitness goals become knockout victims of subconscious desires?
- Where exactly do we draw the line between corporate industries' emotional manipulations and our personal health responsibilities?
- Is the USA culture of "reward and deserve" unique to our obesity-related health complications? How are other countries managing?
- Do men have greater challenges in our outlooks towards fitness? How do those outlooks change in the weight room versus a group class?

- Does our ingrained cultural disdain for "Fat People" show up in the biometrics used to measure our health?
- How soon will the economics of obesity overrun federal and state budgets?
- What corporate entities can help us reverse our obesity trends?

As a prelude to each topic, we'll examine personal, professional, and historical stories. These narratives not only contribute to our understanding of our current societal obesity dilemma but also serve as parallel or contrasting ideologies to the subject matter unique to that chapter.

This book is an investigation into how emotional intelligence can assist the health and fitness industries of our country one person at a time. Not merely what we can do to reverse the alarming trend of health disorders and disease stemming from the declining fitness we've displayed during the last century and into this one; But to assist in being proactive and not reactive within our health care system. We will discuss data and timelines – call them deadlines if you will – for our country's resources.

We will bridge the gap between psychology and our world of fitness to explore the impact on the systems of healthcare.

We'll discuss the cultural and subliminal impact of specific systems in our nation. Those systems for our discussion will be exactly the ones that came to mind on that drive from Philadelphia:

- The fitness industry
- The food and restaurant industry
- Our vast entertainment galaxy
- My insider experiences within the pharmaceutical, research academic, lab diagnostic and distributer industries.

Each system has a specific effect on our collective and individual struggles with obesity.

We'll examine how much money we spend on diets and gyms versus how much money our government spends on our obesity-related illnesses. Is any of that money being spent helping our national obesity issues?

We will review the huge cultural stigmas, pros and cons of psychological counseling, meditation, sleep training and affirmations.

Chapters begin with anecdotes celebrating current and former colleagues and customers from fitness settings, physician offices and research labs that I've witnessed and worked with through the years. We'll even hit the buffet on a cruise.

There are many fantastic individuals who are truly dedicated to driving our country along towards the destinations of health and wellness. We'll continue to need your help, in addition to counseling therapists and emotional-support gurus.

Also, cheers to all those who have tried repeatedly to reach their ultimate fitness goals. We'll all find a way to make this work.

As we'll see from the pages of this book, we literally have no choice.

But first:

Am I an Expert?

Why should anyone listen to me?

I am not a psychologist. My doctorate in Molecular Genetics & Computational Chemistry within a Pharmaceutical & Biomedical Sciences curriculum did not groom me whatsoever to hold discussions on the subconscious mind. Alas, the seven years I spent doing bench-top, biochemical research was within the industries of biotech firms and academia. Those industries most assuredly did not catalyze any discussions on emotional intelligence. Nineteen years on teams exploring testing & therapeutics in the fields of oncology, auto-immune disease, and virology was not a direct steppingstone to the disciplines of psychology, sociology, or public health.

However, almost three decades of employment combined in biotech, academia and as a representative for various large health care and scientific corporations had me working while sitting directly next to *you* in the waiting room of your doctor's office. Which then enabled me to have conversations with your specialty or primary care physicians – while soaking in a spectacular spectrum of socio-economic populations in various healthcare facilities.

Day by day, I spent years discussing the latest trends in biotechnology with those developing as well as implementing those applications. Week by week, I've had an infinite number of exchanges with medical billing specialists while supporting them during their attempts at insurance gymnastics to get the right medications and tests ordered for you, their patient.

Month by month, I've done business presentations to the administrators in the corporate meeting rooms of your local and regional hospitals systems. Year by year, I've spent an overlapping decade as a fitness instructor and personal trainer for circuit weight training facilities and Bikram hot yoga/Pilates studios. You want a great workout directly from me in a group class setting? Put your name on the list!

That drive from Philadelphia to DC put all these experiences from Bikram to the bench top to the boardroom to the bench press towards trying to solve the equation:

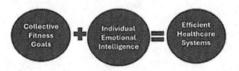

SECTION 2

Explore S.A.M.

CHAPTER 2

How S.A.M. drives
our decisions

THE CHOICES WE MAKE ARE NOT BY ACCIDENT

October 2019. Interstate 95 South.

Two things were occurring on that October drive from Philadelphia to DC:

One. My focus. Obviously, it wasn't completely on the highway. I was highly distracted by the events of that conference and all the domino-effect concepts falling into my mind. Distracted driving is a key point on its own to Explore: The ability to split our attention. How do any of us operate an automobile - at high speeds - while simultaneously picturing the ideas in our heads? Even though my eyes stayed on the road, my mind was engaged in connecting the dots between that conference and our country's fitness issues.

Two: The underlying motivation for me. The issue of fitness and wellness and corporate America had a much bigger scope. My subconscious – without me being fully aware of it, was reaching for its own desires. I was connecting the way people see getting that cheek swab test to *my own journey* with fitness. I had never *fully* reached the fitness levels I attempted to reach.

Whether we're physically driving on a busy interstate or not, our subconscious constantly directs us to make *it* happy. Rarely do we spend our time contemplating any simple or complex idea without a solution that benefits us in *some* capacity. Our subconscious has deeper-seeded desires.

Example: Getting "in shape". How many times do we attempt to get into a workout routine or "give it another try" to lose weight, only to still end up doing, eating, drinking indulging in the same activities that got us overweight in the first place?

Literally it seems someone else is driving us to the fast-food spot we like instead of taking us to the gym.

It seems that as soon as a few days (if we're focused, a few weeks) go by, our new-found zest to change our eating habits or workout routines fades. Our old eating habits come right back.

New diets routinely come and go for us. New gyms, hot yoga, combination workouts and fitness fads come and go.

It's not just that our weight doesn't change, it's that our individual frustrations grow.

Something else is driving our desires and outcomes.

If we literally had to get in the car and drive to "healthier" choices and found ourselves constantly buckled into the passenger seat of the car being driven to eating locations, bars, and "unhealthy" isles in the grocery store, we'd be disturbed.

But that's approximately the narrative happening for many of us. Our Subconscious Autonomous Mind (SAM) is always searching for ways to make itself happy.

SAM is always attempting to do the proverbial driving. It ventures towards all the destinations it deems will make it "happy". It also seeks the comfort and company of people who will acquiesce to its whims.

The delicate conversation topic: How we are frequently just "riding shotgun"; the term for being present in the passenger seat of the car. It's delicate because we all would like to think we're in complete control of our actions and emotions, when frequently our motivations we're not aware of our subconscious' manipulations.

Not only is your subconscious doing the driving, but it *also allows you to feel you're the one behind the steering wheel of the car* - of your decisions. This manifests itself in the maddening whiplash of trying to break your non-fitness habits and then winding back in the cycle of behaviors you were trying to cease.

Emotional Intelligence seeks to understand our subconscious' desires, which frequently interfere with our conscious wants and needs.

The REDI Network creates a discussion platform for delicate topics.

This chapter is **E**xamining how the life choices we make aren't always an accident. Conscious versus our Subconscious.

Our Conscious Mind:

Is Logical & Rational.

Views Time as Linear.

Distinguishes reality from imaginary easily.

Exists to interact with the physical world.

Controls willpower and decision making.

Our Subconscious Autonomous Mind (SAM):

> Does not need to be rational.
> Does not comprehend linear time.
> Struggles to differentiate reality from imaginary.
> Stores all beliefs, habits, and emotions.

On your quest for fitness, SAM functions and processes information & emotions differently – and often in direct conflict - than you do, consciously. If SAM is driving you to destinations that go against your goals, we have a clearer understanding of where the conflict arises.

Here are **6** Ways that SAM conflicts with our fitness desires. We'll get to three in this chapter, on how we battle with SAM every day. In the next chapter, we'll dive into how SAM sees us.

For now, the first three.

1. SAM isn't rational. The constant internal battle between the goals you want and what you wind up not reaching can be frustrating.
2. SAM doesn't understand linear time.
3. SAM truly struggles with what's imaginary versus real.

1: SAM isn't Rational

"Our five senses produce 11 million bits of information per second. Only 40 bits per second are passed on to the Neo-Cortex for conscious processing (thinking, planning etc.). That means that 99.9% of all information from our five senses is only subconsciously processed. The conscious mind is logical, whereas the subconscious mind is imaginal. An imaginal mind builds stories and the stories do not need to be factual." (Goswami, 2012)

As much as we think of ourselves as rational people with a tendency to be logical, SAM is completely the opposite. Our cravings for calorie-heavy, nutrient-deficient foods - or cravings for drugs, sex, relationship enablers, gambling, at levels that aren't healthy for us - are derived from frequently occurring irrational emotions originating from our subconscious.

It doesn't have to make sense at all.

Frequently, that's what baffles and perplexes us when *we know* what we should do and are still unable to consistently execute our plans. We wind up literally and figuratively at places where we *know* we don't need to be.

2: SAM and Linear Time

We can think back and *visit* the past in our minds like arriving at a destination on a map. We can easily go back to our time in 4th or 9th grade or our high school graduation. Our first job. First time we had a crush. That one person we should never have been dating in the first place.

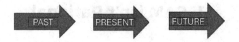

We also can visit times in our past when we endeavored to lose weight or get fit. We know we tried a certain diet and a certain type of exercises, and we retained that we lost - all the weight we wanted to lose, some of the weight, or none of it.

We can make plans for future weight loss. We're going to hit the gym or do hot yoga, or we'll do more walking in the neighborhood.

Except our subconscious has no idea what we're talking about when you talk to it about our ideas of "future plans".

We clash with SAM because it wants what it wants right now!

When we're speaking with SAM about diet plans that include losing weight and what we'll look like 6 months from now? It interprets that as us babbling-on incoherently about imaginary ideas and places.

The real application for this time-paradox: when we're trying to sacrifice having our favorite ice cream or alcoholic beverage for the long-term goal of losing weight over six months, SAM says: *What exactly is a: "Six-Months"? Is that a new sports bar? A new flavor of ice cream?"*

Not only does it *not* comprehend our plans for *"the future"*, but it also holds items *we* view in the past as current and ongoing. It lives every experience in the present.

Example: for all the things we might have *been* through in life:

- dysfunctional household in our youth,
- a difficult romantic breakup,
- fired from a job,

SAM lingers on any of them as if they are still happening in the present.

Our conscious mind views all those things when they occurred in linear time fashion. The breakup was 2 years ago. The job firing was 6 years ago. Our youth was *way back then*. Your subconscious is living it all now. Not yesterday. Now. And unless those items have been resolved to its satisfaction, it will persist on driving to destinations that it desires. Those destinations are its attempts to feel better about *those* situations.

We consciously may think: *"Oh that's been so long ago, I'm over it."* And we can ask that of the people around us – to get over their issues after a certain amount of time has passed. The more time that goes by, the more we're all supposed to be "over" it. Well, the more we wind up at destinations (literal or figurative) that sabotage our "goals", the more we can ask the *questions* about things in our subconscious past that manifest in our current lives.

Questions like:

- Am I out at that bar longer than I wanted to be, even when my husband and kids are asking me to come home? I can consciously justify that I do things for them *all the time* that this is just time for myself. But what is really driving these actions from my childhood?
- I can do all the things necessary to lose weight, but *do I really want to*? Do I really want or deserve all the extra attention I'll get when I'm "in-shape"? Maybe I didn't feel like I deserved attention when I was a child, but I didn't get it.

3: SAM: Reality versus Imagination

It's movie time. You can either go to a movie theater or watch one at home on the couch.

From the safety of your seat in the cinema or couch at home, you are consciously aware that this film is entertainment - not a documentary. It's a fictious, creative artistic expression resplendent with actors, directors, whole camera crew and maybe a special effect editing team.

While you consciously *know* this, you still *jump* when the killer leaps out suddenly from that creepy closet in the bedroom. You still feel the tension of hand-to-hand combat between the hero and the villain in that final fight scene. You still feel the love as the couple who have been not able to fully connect all movie, finally get together in the climactic ending of that romantic comedy.

A well-crafted movie engages our senses as if we directly participated in the story. That's what makes it entertaining! (Or what makes the movie bad if we couldn't connect with the characters or storyline.)

Your subconscious struggles to distinguish between reality and imagination. Yes of course *you* can; because you're logical and rational like point #1.

Your goals of being in shape? Do you fully believe them? Maybe you consciously want it. But deep down do you really want to make sacrifices and keep the discipline to stay out of your comfort foods & beverages for long stretches of time to achieve this task? Your subconscious can't tell. It doesn't know what is real versus what you're just dreaming of, like some movie.

Do you genuinely believe you are going to make it through those *initial* workouts when you're not in shape enough (cardio or strength wise) to even HAVE a good workout? Better question: Do you fully believe you can do *all* the things you need to juggle to reach your goal?

If you don't enjoy the gym, or eating salads, or absorbing all the information of what to eat and when to eat it, or not eating your favorite meals or eating smaller portions *of* those meals, then your subconscious will see all those plans as imaginary.

The movie producers, directors and actors go through a ton of effort to make their product look and feel real. Even when aliens are battling flying superheroes in capes, our subconscious cannot tell that this isn't real, and we feel enthralled and entertained by the time the credits roll up.

Do you really believe that there is a man who turns green from rage, expands muscles so hard he rips completely out of his shirt and then pummels aliens from another dimension – while also keeping his pants on is truly real? It sounds ridiculous and makes me chuckle when I type it. But movies like that make billions of dollars from entertaining our subconscious.

Back to fitness: Do you really believe that this salad, with barely any dressing is going to make up for *not* eating delectable pizza and wings from your favorite delivery place - while also going to the gym is going to work?

What you believe and accept and what your subconscious believes and accepts are two different things.

SAM can't tell the movie is *not* real, but it also can't tell that your desires to lose weight *are* real.

If this discussion concerning psychological materiality becomes as confusing or conflicting as viewing superheroes fighting aliens, then excellent! That's due to your subconscious not exhibiting rationality... it's not trying to help you make sense of this.

You're the one that wants everything to make sense all the time.

We'll come back to that drive from Philadelphia to DC in later chapters. We'll have to go overseas for a bit and go further back in time than just 2019. We'll Examine the findings of a European biologist to help us transition into answering the question: how does SAM see us?

CHAPTER 3

How S.A.M. sees us

FAR STRONGER, IT ALLOWS US TO THINK WE'RE IN CONTROL

1668. Florence, Italy.

In a groundbreaking experiment, a soon-to-be-renowned parasitologist divided six jars into two groups.

Group one had open jars. In group two, the jars were sealed. All the jars contained either raw fish or veal. This scientist published his findings with the title: *Experiments on the generation of insects.* His experiments debunked the theory of Spontaneous Generation.

Fast forward from the 1600s to the upcoming July on your calendar.

You are the host of summer backyard cookout. After everyone has had a plate or two of ribs, chicken and steak, there's still meat exposed on the main table. You go over to cover up the meat because on a hot summer day like today, the flies will be drawn towards it.

Specifically, why do you care about flies alighting on your culinary creations?

It's not as if the flies will consume up all the remaining ribs or zoom off with the chicken. But flies have germs on them, after all they could have just been lingering on the dog poop in the neighbor's yard.

Germs - more specifically bacteria - can multiply rapidly with a nutrient source like your food and either spoil the food with overgrowth or make me, you, and the rest of your guests sick if we ingest it. Also, flies can lay their eggs on the food – leading to a non-tasty development of maggots if left unchecked.

So, it's the bacteria and the dipteran eggs you're protecting us from, not necessarily the flies themselves.

For most of human history, none of us could conceptualize the existence of microscopic organisms - much less how they can spoil our food.

The scientific community *kind of knew* they existed, but our brightest minds in that era couldn't pinpoint their origins. We used to believe that the food (our seasoned venison at the July 1667 renaissance-era cookout) could manifest the growth of other life forms by itself, which was the concept described as: Spontaneous Generation.

The scientist in this story was named Francesco Redi. He challenged that concept.

The R.E.D.I. acronym is not a coincidence. It is a small homage to this 1600s biologist (and creative writer) who is credited with challenging the theories of his era. How he did it was simple. With the sealed jars, he used a *control* group.

In those open jars, he exposed meat to flies as one test. It's not a surprise to us today, but it was a mild shock to folks in the 1600s that meat *not* exposed to flies did *not* develop microscopic larvae leading to visible-to-the-eyes younger flies.

And that application of a control test was greater to the scientific community than merely finding out that insects laying eggs on food leads to maggots.

In the same magnitude of human discovery: The application of being aware of our subconscious emotions is greater than merely applying it to our fitness goals or our obesity crises.

The delicate topic is that we see evidence that our subconscious is at work, but we're not aware of how SAM drives so much of our decision making. It's tough to describe the frustration that we should be able to use our willpower to overcome all the food we ate at that cookout and manifest our fitness aspirations consciously.

The REDI Network creates a discussion platform for delicate topics.

Chapter 3 is here to Examine how our subconscious drives us into choices it wants while allowing us to think we're in control. Self-Awareness.

Here's how SAM sees us:

Out of those 6 ways SAM interferes with our fitness desires, here are those next three items:

1. SAM is far more powerful of an "operating system" for us when compared to our conscious mind.
2. SAM relates everything back to emotions and habits, not facts and information.
3. Our Childhood. SAM is still reliving it in many ways.

1: SAM is More Powerful

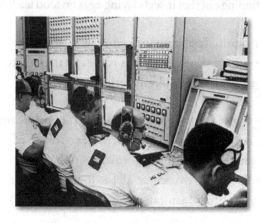

"In 1969 we flew to the moon. Thousands of technicians and computer engineers used the latest technology: The IBM System 360 Model 75s. It was about the size of a car and could communicate between earth and the Lunar astronauts, monitor the spacecraft's environmental data as well as the health of its passengers." (Puiu, 2020)

At the time it was highly impressive: Computers that helped us fly to the moon! Within that article from ZmeScience.com, the author went on to compare those Apollo IBM systems to the computing power of an iPhone6.

In the late 1960s, those Apollo computers were the most complex software ever developed. Today, even a Wi-Fi router is more powerful than those mainframes, let alone a smart phone. From that article, the clock on the iPhone6 is 32,600 times faster than the best Apollo era computers.

That article didn't compare conscious mind to the subconscious, but the comparison is apt. In fact, the power of our subconscious is more than just an iPhone versus a 1969 Apollo computer. The gap is far more substantial.

How substantial? Please allow my biology background to elaborate. Our subconscious regulates all our molecular biology reactions 24 hours a day. Do you personally have time to decide whether to upregulate a specific gene to create more glucose from your gluconeogenesis pathway to avoid hypoglycemia? You don't because your neurological focus is translating the words in this paragraph into functional comprehension.

Well, some entity must monitor those molecular reactions and make an almost infinite amount of proteomic and cellular decisions in *real time*. Not six months from now, not 6 years ago. Right now. Just to keep you alive.

Its computing power holds every single event we ever witnessed, person we met, action we ever took and conversation we ever had in a storage database called memory. When you're supposed to be "over" some traumatic experience because your conscious mind determined (in a rational, linear timeline mindset) that a requisite amount of time has passed? Your subconscious is connecting and compiling *this* recent traumatic event *with all the other events like it* in its exacting memory. And it's irrational – meaning it connects those memories to emotions and beliefs whether warranted or not. In addition, it only sees time as now - it's all happening now!

And you? It's hard for you to remember what you had for breakfast yesterday.

While we're on the subject, let's get back to you. The conscious person reading this sentence. You know what SAM needs from you? It needs physical contact with the material world that you provide. It needs you to matriculate towards the refrigerator freezer and get it more ice cream. Or hold the door open while it scans for what it wants. If you find yourself holding that door open for longer than you anticipated it's because SAM was continuing that argument it was having with a coworker - until you politely remind it to focus back on the wide-open refrigerator door.

SAM needs you to speak into the microphone at the drive through and then physically reach for the food from the cashier. It needs you to physically grasp your smart phone so it can be emotionally entertained on social media and/or get more attention.

It just needs an interface to get what it wants *when* it wants it – which is always in the present time. Now!

Underestimating the power of the subconscious is one of the bigger hurdles we face in terms of understanding our own actions as individuals.

SAM is more powerful than a smart phone. And again, we are the 1969 Apollo computers, we're only impressive for the limited number of tasks we're capable of doing.

How did this end up this way? Well, our subconscious evolved this way centuries ago. It was created to handle the emotions of the physical world we live in. Throughout our human history, it has kept us safe to not stray away from things we know by reminding us of potential danger: fear of the unknown.

It double checks to make sure there's not a bear past that bend in the trail that we can't see around. That's in addition to its task of keeping us physically alive with millions of micro-tasks we'd never be able to keep track of on our own.

SAM is a sophisticated, high-powered operating system. It becomes easily overlooked because not only do we view the *same* images it *does* out of the front seat, but it also allows us to believe we're the ones driving.

2: Beliefs, Emotions, Habits

The analogy of driving a car goes back to the original drive from Philadelphia to DC after that conference. However, due to the contentious nature of our conscious goals vs our subconscious desires, the more appropriate analogy would be more akin to a fight.

A Boxing Match.

In one corner, we're going to use our conscious "willpower" to throw punches and use our decision making to avoid getting hit. That is, using our 1969 computing power we resolve to finally to lose weight and get fit.

Those conscious goals are opposed in the match by our opponent across the ring from us: SAM.

Our conscious has been working hard its whole life creating our habits, forming our beliefs, compiling our emotions by entering and storing all the information it's ever seen or heard or been exposed in our lifetime. How does SAM see you? It's seen and experienced every single detail about you.

Beliefs. SAM doesn't just store the beliefs we have about politics or sports or religion or relationships – those are in there as well – but about the beliefs of ourselves and our own capabilities.

Emotions. It doesn't just store the fractured or full emotional attachments we have to our loved ones but also emotions we are still struggling to seed, water and grow. Remember, it only sees time as the present, it's actively trying to work on any trauma we've ever experienced in the present moment.

Habits. It's been working on our habitual routines and comfort zones since we were born with every bit of emotional and physical data up to and including this day.

Contrast that with your knowledge of it. You may not have even heard of your opponent for this boxing match. Much less studied SAM's techniques. You don't know its moves; how hard it hits. You're going to try and punch your way through all that with what you figure can get you through: Will Power.

Good luck. Because the *one* thing SAM has been studying this whole time is you!

It knows all your "rational" moves. The things you try and tell yourself about what you want to "accomplish". It ducks all your punches, no matter how hard you swing. It absolutely knows you haven't been training for it. It can handle the "Power" of your Will-punches easily. It moves much faster than your Decision Making. It throws punches from angles you can't see coming. It's not a fair fight. You'll last a few rounds (which means you'll last a few days or weeks with your new "dedication" to your fitness goals). If you haven't trained for it, you'll be forced to throw in the towel.

So that's all six? Not yet. There is one more.

Going back to our centuries of human development, we needed our willpower so that we didn't eat our crops or livestock before they finished growing. We understood the concept of time so that we could, among other things, plan our harvest and remember that in the past, the rainy season would bring more moisture to our lands. All of that only requires 5% to 10% of our minds.

Now that getting access to food or growing it from seeds to harvest isn't an issue. Now that being eaten by a bear isn't a worry or concern:

- Our childhood becomes a concern.
- Our career path is a concern.
- Our love-life is a concern.
- And our super-computer-chip subconscious is all-in on making itself feel better about those things – first. That is the priority!

Before we leave this chapter, we've got one additional deeper dive. Our Childhood.

3.Our Childhood

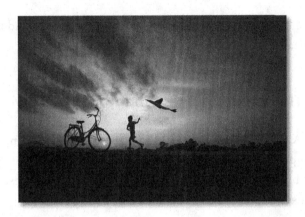

"Exposure to stressful events in childhood can increase the impact of stressful events throughout life. It seems how you cope with stressful experiences is not only influenced by your prior experiences, but also your genes, coping responses and brain regulation." (Baracz, 2018)

To varying extents, we're all still grappling to get over what happened to us (or didn't happen, like nurturing) in our youth. Academic research has shown it isn't just purely our long-term emotions that are affected. Our brain hormones are affected by stress versus nurture in our youth.

From a counselor perspective, so many issues that motivate adults into counseling have an original source created in our childhood.

"Experiencing trauma as a child can lead to a host of emotional and psychological issues that may not emerge until later in life. Adults who experienced trauma during childhood may experience difficulties in many aspects of their lives. They may not realize that these traumatic experiences are contributing factors to their current issues or even the root cause of them." (DualDiagnosis.org)

We're largely *unaware* of these issues we have we derive from our childhood. Or we're minimizing the effect it has on our adult lives.

"Adverse childhood experiences are the single greatest unaddressed public health threat facing our nation today." (Block)

The impact our childhood has on SAM:

Since SAM doesn't understand the concept of linear time, SAM can compare it's needs to correct adverse childhood events versus what is being proposed to it by our conscious in the present. It's asking us:

> "You really want to lose weight? I'm not really worthy of a great body/physique."

> Or:

> "I don't really want to do all those sacrifices of food and workouts and research."

> Or:

> "I'm scared of changing."

"Every person who has walked through my door suffering from depression, anxiety, relationship or work problems, low self-esteem or addiction has a history of some type of adversity in their childhood. It's becoming clear to me by listening to their stories that were it not for these painful events, the person would not be struggling as much as they are today." (Sirota)

Allow me to venture back to the beginning of the book. That conference in Philadelphia. It's SAM that drives the irrational fear of getting that check swab test. All that SAM is concerned about is the present potential in maintaining habits. It will not give up things it likes without a boxing match. It strives to constantly "feel better" about itself.

So, in that moment when someone proposes taking a test for a rare genetic disorder, it quickly counters with information that would make it unwise to visit the doctor's office. Our rational brain makes up some excuse to agree with it to not have to have an internal boxing match and we move on. Or rather, we stay the same.

These internal conflicts are seen even more versus the various industries that manipulate our subconscious.

CHAPTER 4

USA fitness and obesity

SAM VERSUS THE FOOD & RESTAURANT INDUSTRIES

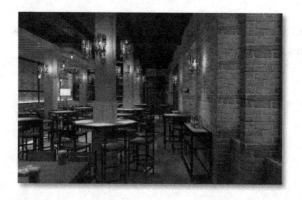

Spring 2021. Washington, DC.

Since the original March 2020 shutdown, it's now been 14 months of quarantine with no gym workouts, no hot Pilates, no hot yoga. Just walking in the neighborhood when the weather was decent. I was as out of shape as I had ever been in my adult life.

Allow me to be 100% honest. I have never been obese. Not even overweight. I'm usually in slightly-better-than-average condition cardio and strength-wise for a middle-aged human. And even after those 14 months, my frame was just lacking muscle tone as opposed to having high body fat % or any developed health risks.

The point is: Even without that life-as-we-know-it-altering Viral Quarantine, I've still had my own personal struggles through the decades *giving up* the *one* thing that used to keep me from being in excellent/elite shape. And it wasn't anything related to the SARS-C0V-2 virus.

It was The Bar Scene.

The journey to my own self-awareness involved asking the question: What is it about going to bars that made me *so willing* to stay in that scene despite it being contrary to my fitness goals? I even had a fitness mentor (the lead personal trainer at the now-defunct Bally's Total Fitness chain of gyms) constantly imploring with me to abandon the bar scene – for just two or three months - to see the maximum results from our weight-lifting sessions.

But I stayed in that scene periodically enough to neutralize my otherwise stellar fitness activities. I stayed in neutral. Not overweight, in "decent" shape, but not in elite fitness like I claimed I wanted to be.

What were the reasons? I can't make this statement clear enough: It wasn't just the alcohol itself in those bars. I could make my own drinks at home (and I almost *never* drink at home by myself).

It wasn't just bar food. If I weren't having a drink there, I wouldn't even have one fleeting thought of their food menus.

It was the ambiance of sports bars. It was the pizzaz of trendy bars. The aristocracy of upscale lounges. The sunny tranquility of a tiki bar. The marvelous cozy dilapidation of dive bars.

The diversity of the atmospheres fed into my subconscious desires to socialize with a broad spectrum of people. The fact that I could get a drink *made for* me (and sure why not, maybe even some food) made my subconscious feel all-grown-up-and-stuff.

Pushing the vulnerability limits further into my childhood, which was great *inside* the walls of the house where I grew up. But outside that house? The 80s and 90s crack epidemic turned my native DC into a shooting gallery with hustlers and addicts all vying to create an urban warzone that I struggled to adapt as a teen. Specifically, my upbringing as a proper-speaking, nerdy naiveté did not blend in with the cut-throat, face-paced "hood mentality" in which many American big cities in that era were embroiled. So, to not become an easy target in a hostile environment, I became bilingual and dual-cultural – quickly (fluent Ebonics and vibrationally urban).

Sitting at the bar sipping a drink (on a date, with friends or solo) made me cool. Period.

Applying different decibels and wavelengths from my cultural arsenal to camouflage perfectly with the assortment of bartenders and bar patrons in their native settings was a bonus.

Is any of that rational – the connection to childhood insecurities being soothed by the social proving grounds of bars? Of course not, especially *versus* my adult long-standing, conscious fitness goals.

Is it individualized for just me and my subconscious? Yes and no.

No, in the sense that I'm obviously not the only one present in these establishments. But yes - in the sense that everyone else's internal reasons for frequenting the bar scene are completely unique, and we're all getting some satisfaction from it subconsciously.

And that feeling – that satisfaction my SAM got from socializing at some fantastically extravagant - or brilliantly dilapidated - bar was well worth going against my conscious desire for being in elite fitness condition.

Another enormously contradictory point I need to make clear for a full discussion on fitness journeys: I am always eager to workout. Lifting at the gym or running on the local high-school track or taking/teaching hot Pilates/yoga never required one bit of "discipline" from me. I enjoy all aspects and angles of working out, consciously and subconsciously. No internal boxing matches when it comes to exercise.

Still staying honest and still staying on the topics of fitness and obesity: I'll also eat *relatively* healthily when I'm fixing food at home (and not physically at the bar or restaurant, where I might eat whatever looks delicious to my SAM). I don't crave snacks or sweets (via genetics, my apologies to those that do). I'll eat great pre-and-post-workout meals. I'll stay hydrated.

No problem!

But give up the bar? For weeks or months?

Give up Happy Hour in the major metropolitan cities, or small college towns where I've lived and can be Mr. Cosmopolitan/ Man-about-town?

Problem!

Again, only through self-reflection after researching to write these books, I now realize it's never strictly been about the drinks & alcohol themselves. Previously, I would have sworn that I just love social drinking. Now I see just how much lighting and music and chair arrangements were keeping me going back to certain environments. And I see why I rarely drank at the house – my subconscious liked the *environments* created by these establishments, which just happened to have beer, wine, and cocktails.

I had no idea of the full scope of how I was being emotionally manipulated, and it all makes sense now.

But it's not just my personal *"bar calories versus workout routines"* that knocks down the dominoes for this book (or more specifically for these next two chapters).

It's those two decades years in the pharmaceutical and lab diagnostic industries, walking in and out of doctors' offices and hospitals for a living. I witness how much money and effort we spend *after* we've become sick from whatever ailments occur not only from our obesity (a lot) but from our stress levels and overall lack of being healthy and happy.

Those seven additional years spent on the bench top in biotech and academia, I was diligently working with some of the best scientific minds in our field on developing treatments that could help *reactively.* That is to say: post-infection, post-trauma, post-disease-state-diagnosis.

Our focus in health care rarely is taken up proactively, much less do we attempt to battle the individual wars with ourselves versus these various industries.

The REDI Network creates a discussion platform for delicate topics.

Chapter 4 is here to **E**xamine the emotional manipulation of
The Food Manufacturing
Industry versus SAM

Fitness Goals Versus Corporate America

So now that we know how our subconscious can work against us in our fitness journeys, how does SAM see the world around us? More specifically, how does our subconscious battle the various corporate industries and systems in our country?

In the United States, we juggle and throw money at an assortment of workout facilities, more varieties of diets than days in the year, and a ton of studies, health care professionals and internet fitness experts all weighing in on how to lose weight and stay healthy. It seems *impossible* that with all these resources we'd still be overweight.

However, it's more than possible. It's reality. If you're feeling like you need to lose a few pounds (or more than a few) you aren't the only one in the country feeling that way. The United States is one of the *least healthy* (which is *such* a nice phrase for "fat") nations on earth. How "fat" are we in comparison to other obese countries around the world?

COUNTRY	World Rank	% of population obese
Nauru	#1	61.00%
Cook Islands	2	55.9
Palau	3	55.3
Marshall Islands	4	52.9
Tuvalu	5	51.6
Niue	6	50.0
Tonga	7	48.2
Samoa	8	47.3
Kiribati	9	46.0
Federated States of Micronesia	10	45.8
Kuwait	11	37.9
United States	12	36.2
Jordan	13	35.5
Saudi Arabia	14	35.3
Qatar	15	35.1

(Agency, 2017)

A further look at the 11 countries with a higher percentage than us reveals: Ten of the eleven nations ranking ahead of the USA for percentage are small islands in the Pacific Ocean. Kuwait, at 37.9% is the only non-island nation that had a higher percentage of obese people.

We do indeed consciously *believe* we need to be in better shape, or we wouldn't be spending significant portions of our collective incomes on trying to change our waistlines via gyms and diets.

In the previous two chapters, we went over 6 ways SAM impedes our thinking towards losing weight. This chapter we'll cover four industries that are communicating directly with our subconscious. Those industries are seeking ways to increase their profits within our capitalistic system. SAM sees each tactic implemented by these industries to capitalize on feeling better about itself.

There are four industries that manipulate SAM. We'll discuss two now. Then the next two in the following chapter.

1. The USA Food Manufacturing Industry

Going back to our international obesity standings. What role does the manufacturing of our food play in these statistics?

"Blame and shame for unhealthy behaviors occur because obesity is often framed as an issue of personal responsibility. In this narrative, we alone are responsible for what goes into our mouths. If we gain weight, it is a result of gluttony, sloth, and lack of willpower." (Daley, 2017)

Are we sure it's not just "us" and our lack of discipline? Before we ask questions on the responsibilities of industries? Are Americans just lazy? Do we lack the restraint to overcome our desires to eat our way near the top of an obese countries list?

In that quote from Beth Daley, we see that word again: "Willpower". Previously we used it to compare our conscious mind being overmatched as a late 1960's computer or in a boxing match. We're not just overmatched against our subconscious. We're taking on this entire industry, and it's not just the quality of the food.

We're not talking about nutritional values or lack thereof. It's not just that the food industry can create cheap and available products which continue to call to us from our cabinets, pantries, refrigerators, and freezers. We're also hard-wired to respond to how delicious food has become. We're literally salivating to get more delectable food. And this industry is aware of the biological effects their products have on our psyches.

"Salivation is part of the experience of eating food, and the more a food causes you to salivate, the more it will swim throughout your mouth and cover your taste buds. For example, emulsified foods like butter, chocolate, salad dressing, mayonnaise and ice cream promote a salivary response that helps to lather your taste buds with goodness. This is one reason why so many people enjoy foods that have sauces or glazes on them. The result is that foods that promote salivation do a happy little tap dance on your brain and taste better than ones that don't." (Clear)

Two things stood out from that quote: Salad dressing and "enjoy".

Whether or not we start eating the stereotypical salads to lose weight, the dressing we put on can negate every bit of calorie reduction we're aiming for – and still have us hooked on it!

But primarily, foods can be manufactured to create not just taste but psychological enjoyment.

"Dynamic contrast refers to a combination of different sensations in the same food. Foods with dynamic contrast have "an edible shell that goes crunch followed by something soft or creamy and full of taste-active compounds. This rule applies to a variety of our favorite food structures — the caramelized top of a creme brulee, a slice of pizza, or an Oreo cookie — the brain finds crunching through something like this very novel and thrilling." (Clear)

James Clear goes on to detail even how foods are designed to tantalize our taste buds (and our brain) in ways we're not thinking about.

Why? Because great tasting food leads to pleasure and *pleasure* is a reward for the subconscious's insatiable desire to feel better about itself!

Even when we prepare food at home, we attempt to make our food as delicious as possible to emulate the delicious food we crave from the food industry. SAM sees food as a grand occasion to gain enjoyment from, not as sustenance for biological survival. If your food is not pleasing to SAM, it is not going to be happy and in turn, it will make sure you're not "happy".

So, are we infuriated at the food industry? Meaning, are we upset at the people that came up with ideas to create foods that overload our taste senses (and emotions) to be more desirable to us, even if it's not always healthy for us?

Of course not.

"Your brain likes variety. When it comes to food, if you experience the same taste over and over again, then you start to get less pleasure from it. In other words, the sensitivity of that specific sensor will decrease over time. This can happen in just minutes.

Junk foods, however, are designed to avoid this sensory specific. They provide enough taste to be interesting (your brain doesn't get tired of eating them), but it's not so stimulating that your sensory response is dulled. This is why you can swallow an entire bag of potato chips and still be ready to eat another. To your brain, the crunch and sensation of eating Doritos is novel and interesting every time." (Clear)

These corporate entities are finding the best way to maximize the literal consumption of their products. The REDI acronym allows us to be consciously aware of it. SAM already is.

For most of the time we existed on planet Earth, food was just merely a way to stay alive. The last few generations have created a new consequence – eating as an event.

In this country, it's frequently an emotional event sponsored by a corporate entity. And that #12 ranking isn't just driven by the food we crave while we're at home, it's also helped by our next subject: the restaurant industry.

2. Restaurants

For this discussion, separate the food itself from the brick-and-mortar building of a restaurant and focus on the experiences provided inside these businesses. Whether small or large, chain or locally owned, see these facilities as corporate entities that just happen to have digestible products.

That being said. I love restaurants. And as mentioned previously, bars and lounges as well, as they all strive to promote an environment, not just a product. The variety of choices is stunning. From upscale, trendy & posh to The Great American Chains (TGIFridays, Applebee's, Chili's, Ruby Tuesday, you get the idea) to sports bars to ubiquitous fast food.

When you call or text someone about a new restaurant you just visited, you would tell them about the main two things you saw: The food and the service.

If something else was amiss, like the cleanliness wasn't up to par or parking was tough to find, you'll add that.

But SAM had an entirely separate experience.

Restaurants are doing four main things (A, B, C, D) to communicate directly with our subconscious. These four techniques are all outside of what you experience consciously (good customer service and food taste).

A. Restaurant Colors

Restaurants deliberately choose specific colors as part of their interior and exterior décor. If you've never noticed it, previously, neither had my conscious up until this research. Now I see it everywhere.

"Blues, purples, and greens are known as the more difficult restaurant color schemes. The easier color schemes are red, yellow, and orange, and the neutrals: beige, ivory, white, taupe, brown, etc. Warm colors promote positive feelings. They are also more stimulating colors that have been proven to increase one's appetite, so be sure to correctly proportion warm colors and not overpower your food by having red walls and tons of red fixtures in the same room." (Signs.com, 2014)

It's subtle yet effective subconscious emotional manipulation. Restaurants can "increase my appetite" with colors! I was *flabber-and-ghasted* to find this out. Also, from this quote above: Don't "overpower" my food with colors. It's a stunning revelation that warm colors stimulate positive feelings. (Again, *who said SAM was rational?*)

So, my subconscious is absorbing all these things - and more importantly remembering them - so that it can attain those feelings again. Because it remembers everything and doesn't understand linear time, it wants it again, right now.

B. Restaurant Lighting and Windows

The dim lights that establish the ambiance in an upscale restaurant are not a coincidence. Our conscious mind might see it as "atmosphere". But low lighting encourages us to savor our food.

Bright light leads to high turnover, more customers in and out.

Restaurants with both: bright lights at the bar and low lights at their tables want to maximize both effects.

I had to think about it. I've never been to a dimly lit fast-food restaurant.

And neither have you. They do not exist. Fast food restaurants are always bright. The windows all around constantly remind SAM of the places it needs to go next to continue to make itself feel better in the present. The bright lights and windows get us in and out. Fast food and fast customers. Fast food goliaths like McDonalds, Burger King and Subway originated in the USA and while they've expanded globally, it's so much seen as American culture than other countries see it as the Americanization of their cultures. There is no corner of our vast country that is void of our Burgers, Wings, Pizza, and sugary sodas.

Back to lighting itself: Higher priced restaurants can be dimly lit for the environment they create within the space. We stay longer to order *additional* high-priced items from their menu. You've never seen a dimly lit fast-food place just like you've never seen a high-end restaurant have a drive-through. The lack of windows in a posh establishment (and casinos) leads SAM to want to *stay put for a while* and run up a nice high bill. Because SAM is having such a good time (if this all plays into its comfort zone) it will convince the conscious mind that this won't count *too much* against the diet you've been trying to maintain.

Personal Story: I used to complain that one of my very favorite large restaurants/bars - just east of Washington, DC - didn't have any windows. I thought it would be nice even if they built a sunroof, a deck, or something to even *see* outside. I knew they could afford to do it because the place is always packed. *Now I see why it's always packed.* And additionally, I see why I gravitate toward this corporate entity myself - *because it has no windows*!

It allows SAM to be completely focused on staying in there for hours (which my friends and I always do and we're frequently repeat customers). And this is despite their food being mostly just "ok" and to the blunt, their customer service frequently "less than ok". That restaurant does a masterful job of communicating with SAM.

C. Restaurant Music

Whether it's live or over the sound system: If its slow tempo and soothing? Diners stay longer and are more prone towards having a higher bill.

Fast music? Up-tempo? Patrons get in and out quickly and profits are maximized by getting as many people in and out as possible.

D. Restaurant Spacing

People subconsciously feel more uncomfortable sitting in the middle of the restaurant, so if that's where the restaurant wants more turnover, that's where they'll seat more guests or arrange the table that way. Guests linger longer when they're seated at the perimeter.

Those are four of the ways the restaurant industry communicates with SAM. I can trace back in my own life and say I've been easy prey for manipulations of colors and lighting, windows, and seating arrangements.

The point isn't to delineate which restaurant is executing which subconscious emotional gymnastics on any given dining event. The point is to be conscious enough to know that there is *far more* happening than merely our food and our server. And for the purposes of our fitness journey, we need to recognize that SAM already knows all of this about this industry, and more importantly, the industry has known how to communicate with SAM.

Without that acknowledgement, SAM will continue to drive us to restaurants where we get the food it craves *in addition* to the colors, seating, lighting, and background noise it enjoys. We're just along for the ride.

I was.

Restaurants with full business savvy intentions make SAM feel so much better about itself. Our subconscious mind is relentlessly trying to feel better about itself – your desires to lose weight are sometimes an annoying obstacle.

Amusement parks and luxury hotels resorts sell the same emotions to us. Amusement parks sell fun. Luxury resorts sell relaxation and elegance. If your subconscious loves fun, or seeks relaxation, or adores elegance, you are these corporate entities' target.

Even burgers chains aren't simply cooking delectable burgers to engage our saliva-response, they're marketing how good you're going to feel about yourself while eating it.

To be clear, SAM doesn't just taste the food and feel the ambiance of the restaurants. It absorbs our corporate marketing as well. All the actors in food, beer and restaurant commercials are feeling better about themselves while enjoying these products than you are on your couch. Those people in those commercials are literally jumping off cliffs into tropical water or high-fiving friends in sports bar or relaxing with friends enjoying a picturesque city skyline. They're having a blast.

Versus you. You with all your bills, your health issues, your job that you "tolerate", your friends and family that are occasionally problematic.

You want what those people have in those commercials. Happiness.

Joy. Serenity. Whatever it is you're lacking. And SAM associates all those emotions with all those products.

So, it's general and gentle emotional manipulation in which the food and entertainment industry engages. But our reaction to it and attachment to those entities is still *very much individually* based.

We all have our *unique experiences* via each individual subconscious. And because of those unique life experiences and childhoods, no one has the same two reasons why they don't want to give up their emotional attachment to the things they enjoy: Pasta, a favorite alcoholic beverage, wings, their favorite restaurant etc.

Make no mistake, the food/restaurant industry is speaking to our subconscious directly, sidestepping our conscious along the way.

Are we irate at the restaurant industry?

That's a "no" as well. Nobody wants to take the joy out of dining-out with friends or family. We just want to be aware of what's happening *while* we're enjoying ourselves. Again, this is our system: Make a product. Find some customers. Market and sell that product. Rinse and repeat. We use the ink-pen of self-awareness to draw the line between the restaurant industry's manipulations and our own personal responsibilities.

How we **I**mpact that system/industry is a discussion in our final section. But for now, all this talk about food has me hungry. I know where we can get tons of food at an all-you-can-eat buffet. On a cruise!

All aboard!

CHAPTER 5

USA fitness and obesity

SAM VERSUS THE ENTERTAINMENT INDUSTRY

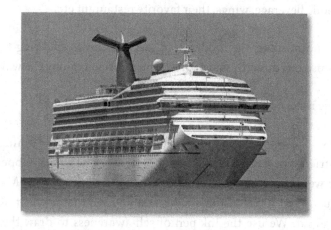

April 2023. Miami Florida.

The security check point lines were longer than I anticipated. It gave me time to think while boarding for my first time ever on a cruise. I actively thought about all the co-workers, family and friends who had told me what to expect once I got onboard.

Most of them said it will be fun because it's Carnival Cruise Lines and those are never stuffy. Everyone mentioned that I'll be lost and turned-around the first few hours/days because the ships are humongous. They said there would be cool, yet touristy destinations at port.

But one person's advice on cruising stood out before and during my cruise experience.

The owner of the Hot Yoga & Hot HIIT Pilates studio where I teach classes had her own perspective about how she was a bit turned off by "all the eating" people do on those cruises. When she shared her perspective days before my cruise, I truly had no idea what she was talking about. I chuckled to myself: "I love to eat; I hope nobody is going to be judging me when I'm stuffing myself on this cruise".

When that studio owner mentioned it, I felt palpable disdain and mild disgust in her voice. That takeaway she shared with me was so real for her, it lasted all the way into me boarding the ship.

I contrasted her take with my other friends and family. When they mentioned "the food", they had the tone that it would be a *great* thing; something to look forward to on my floating vacation. Awesome. I'm ready! All aboard.

Then when I saw it, I couldn't believe it.

Whatever day it is you're reading this, trust me, I am *still* blown away by the sheer amount of my fellow Americans on that cruise who were overweight to obese. I felt …more than sad …. I felt bewildered while watching folks from all over the country (but mainly the South and Midwest) have a blast stuffing themselves around the clock at the buffets.

It's one thing for people to let loose and maybe overeat while on vacation. I planned on doing just that myself. It's another thing when the segment of our population that can least afford to be stuffing themselves – and I mean from a health perspective, not an economic one – are doing just that.

Pause.

(If the terms Body Positivity or Fat Shaming are familiar to you, skip to Chapter 12 right now. We'll meet you *right back here*, I promise. If those terms have no gravity for you, please proceed.)

Now I understood what the Yoga studio owner was trying to encapsulate. It wasn't the food, or the buffet stations themselves. It was the *scene* of who's eating it and how much they're eating.

In sharp contrast to that cruise, four very short months later I went on a vacation on an island off southern Spain. It wasn't my imagination – and it was completely unexpected - that so many people of all ages in Ibiza were lean. In fact, the only "heavy" people we saw for days at a time were the people within my travel group – my fellow Americans.

The REDI Network creates a discussion platform for delicate topics.

Chapter 5 is **E**xamining the emotional manipulation of The Entertainment Industry versus SAM

---

1. Television & Movies affect obesity

We need to transition from the topic of cruising - for now. Let's focus on how a significant portion of our population walks onto that cruise overweight in the first place. This is about our overall emotional attachment to the entertainment industry as a whole and the effect that industry has on obesity and fitness.

Mostly we're talking about a time paradox. Our TV shows and movies compete with not just our conscious versus SAM. It competes with our physical ability to only be in one place at a time.

Alterations might need to be made to our 24-hour-day schedule if we're going to make changes in our habits. Remember, the whole idea for this book, this concept, was a woman who quoted at a conference: "...*people don't want to give up their TV shows*".

It's a comfort zone that is not going to go out quietly if we're trying to change habits to be healthier. Remember SAM doesn't want to give up anything that makes it feel better about itself. We literally can't be in the gym or at the store getting fresh food more often (because fresh food can spoil so quickly) while we're watching TV from our couch.

The Entertainment Industry can be far more than just a time paradox.

Remember our subconscious can't tell the difference between what's real and what's imaginary. So, the entertainment industry works hard with SAM into creating various realities where their shows and movies become important.

We all have different backgrounds of various childhood and life experiences. Shows that appeal to your experiences will be different than mine. The television industry is banking that there is:

- A reality-singing or dancing show that emotionally ties itself to your past desires to be a singer or dancer.
- Sports: You can emotionally attach to your hopes that maybe you could have become a professional athlete. Or sports talk shows that lend themselves towards you wanting to be a sports analyst.

- A crime drama, binge-worthy, streaming-series that brings out elements of your youth growing up in a city – or how you wish you had.
- A situation-comedy that has characters that remind you of you and your friends – or makes you wish you had a supportive circle just like that.
- A movie where the hero is rebellious and free-spirited: doesn't like to be told what to do. Deep down, neither do you.

SAM emotionally attaches itself to *anything* it relates to from its vast memory of events in your lifetime. Are you aware of why you like that show? How hard would it be to give it up or miss it (even if you could record it and watch it later) if some aspect of losing weight required a time conflict (not just with recording the show or binging it on a streaming service, but there are so many hours in a day and the choice may be being entertained versus being in the gym).

SAM emotionally attaches to television as much as it attaches to the lighting & sounds of any restaurant or the deliciousness of saliva-inducing food. SAM sees TV shows/movies/sports as a *real world* in which it can feel better about itself.

2. Social Media

Facebook. Instagram. Tik-Tok. Twitter is now "X". LinkedIn. Their algorithms were originally designed to have us spend as much time as possible on their sites to expose us to as many of their advertisements as possible.

One can *argue* that their effect on SAM is the most manipulative, dangerous influence in the history of technology. But that sounds way too much of a "conspiracy theory" and from many accounts (documentaries such as *"The Social Dilemma", "The Great Hack"*) it was not intentional during its inception.

Still for the purposes of our discussion, it is again, an emotional attachment that can physically eat up minutes and hours in the limited amount of time we have per every 24 hours, when we're attempting to *not* be the #12 ranked obese country on planet earth.

Directly, the time spent commenting and posting on social media could be time we would be comparing diet plans, or the right protein-carbohydrate mix for our particular phase in our workout routines.

For some, taking the time to "sort through" that diet/workout information never happens. Just like the conference in Philadelphia, there are so many resources and information available, one still must take the time to go through it all. Otherwise, it just gets wasted.

Many folks throw up their hands without even attempting to find out what to eat and when – but they don't miss their shows and you can see them frequently posting/commenting on social media.

(Not to mention, for as many people sharing their workout and fitness routines via social media, there are that many people sharing pictures of their delicious food and fun they're having while at some "awesome new" restaurant. You want the workouts. SAM sees all that food!)

Twitter debates with a twinkie in hand versus South Beach Diet reviews with smoothie in the blender? We can only spend so much waking time on our phones. SAM wants to be "entertained" - Now! Do you really *want* to be spending that time researching the caloric and nutritional difference of strawberries vs egg salad for your next grocery store run?

(Or maybe even googling what calories are? We all know the various emoji "like buttons" on Facebook but knowing what a calorie is could help us understand nutrition, right?)

That would be the logical, rational course of action for someone attempting to lose weight, but it doesn't sound like as much *fun* as surfing through Instagram or Tik Tok.

It is your *choice* how you spend your time. Or is SAM doing the driving?

A double setback for our obesity rates is when we're watching television with our favorite foods in front of us. SAM sees that as a wonderful emotional event, a huge reward to itself for putting up with your desires to do "other productive things".

The triple setback is when we turn on our favorite TV event, with our favorite delicious foods in front of us *and* surf social media all simultaneously (maybe even texting our friends as well). You think our 1969 Apollo computer conscious mind can compete with that triple addiction dose that SAM loves? I mean, I'm laughing while I'm typing this sentence because it's not a fair fight.

(Full disclosure again. I am completely guilty of committing this triple dietary felony. I get – that is, I used to get – excited over the idea of The Big Game on TV tonight with my wings and/or sandwich plus dipping sauces and cheese-filled-somethings plus an alcoholic drink while going back and forth about the game on social media or - more likely - in a group text. But what's my emotional attachment to all those segments individually and collectively if I had to give them up to get in elite shape? I mean, I say I want to get in elite shape. Right? Fact is, I already feel my mind justifying how I don't have to give those things up. My mind starts calculating that I can make up for it in some other capacity – eat less the day before – work out harder the next day at the gym – anything besides giving up that triple hit of Football, Favorite Foods, and Facebook.)

So, are we individually and collectively somehow angry with social media companies or with the television/entertainment industry?

The answer is again: No.

All we need to do is be aware of all these factors on a conscious level. These corporations are not collaborating to "sabotage" us from our fitness goals. They're just trying to make money. Again, SAM already knew all this stuff anyway. We're the ones that act like this is all new information.

All Emotional Landmines

Here's how SAM sees all of this:

- Food should always be amazingly scrumptious, every single bite.
- Restaurants are places to go to feel better about itself outside of the food and service.
- Social media and television shows are absolute reality.

None of it is a coincidence that we crave these things. All of it should be brought to our conscious mind that this is what SAM sees and feels.

To be clear for each of us as individuals, it's usually not a long list of things that get in our way on our journey towards physical fitness. The industries we've discussed in this chapter aren't *all* problems for *all* of us. In addition, there are so many things that *we are willing* to do to get in shape.

Our willingness to do several things to help ourselves lose weight conflicts with the small number of issues holding us back. Remember, we might be the #12 obese country on the planet, but with our conscious minds we spend a ton on trying to get fit.

Meaning even more so, those industries we *just* mentioned are not "the villains". They employ us, our friends, our family. Maybe you don't know any computer engineers in Silicon Valley or actors in Hollywood, but everyone knows a waiter or bartender or grocery store employee.

The companies themselves are just attempting to show their stockholders (*Which is us, right? I mean you do hold stocks in these entities/destinations where your subconscious drives you to, correct? Otherwise, you would be just throwing your time and money at them, and who would do that?*) quarter by quarter, year by year returns on investment by increasing revenues while holding expenses steady. That's Business 101.

We understand all that about business. We are the ones that are rational. However, SAM is not the same.

Maybe *you're* not on clear and open speaking terms with your subconscious but these other entities & companies sure are. They are communicating directly with SAM. Those other entities: food and entertainment and social media companies are extremely *aware* of how to direct and manipulate our subconscious; all while we're consciously oblivious.

Wait. This just covers America. What about the rest of the world? All humans have a subconscious. And many countries are struggling with obesity. Some aren't.

Let's look at a few:

Japan: According to the National Institutes of Health (NIH.gov) the 3.5% obesity rate in Japan is one of the lowest in developed countries.

This is attributed to not only their traditional diet that includes fish, whole grains, and vegetables but a culture that promotes portion control and physical activity.

South Koreans think of themselves as overweight. The data sets are indeed conflicting for South Korea, as the Organization for Economic Cooperation and Development (OECD) reports a 5.9% obesity rate while other agencies have this country above 30%. Part of it is what *they consider obese* from a Body Mass Index perspective. In other words, what the USA measures as overweight and South Korea measures as overweight are two different things. However, their diet of fermented foods, lean protein and active lifestyle leads to a culture of fitness awareness. (Nam, 2021)

Switzerland: According to the Swiss Health Survey, between 1992 and 2017 the percentage of obese people in Switzerland doubled from 5% to 11%. The past few years have seen this rate stabilize. The Swiss promote fresh and locally sourced food and a culture of outdoor activities.

In summary, we can't merely attribute the USA obesity crisis to food or entertainment. Our culture, in contrast to other nations, is not one of fitness awareness or physical activity much less portion control. We do indeed have segments of our society that are fitness oriented. We're doing better in our cities promoting bicycle lanes and walking trails (if for no other reason that attempting to cut down on car traffic and fossil fuel emissions, it still leads to increased physical fitness). However, we are still losing the battle versus our corporate America industries advancing food and entertainment to satiate our work-culture collective mentality. That's in addition to our diet being anchored by convenience and leisure.

> We just want to go home and watch our favorite shows on television.

Large segments of our American culture – as witnessed on my Carnival cruise – do not have a fitness orientation. We want continuous eating continuous drinking to be *part of the entertainment* – the topic of this chapter is just as much to do with our outlook on how we "deserve" all you can eat and then lay around in the sun as much as it is about the industries themselves.

In fact, that cruise is a microcosm for how America prioritizes fitness versus being entertained. More specifically: On that ship there was indeed a gym. There was a basketball half court. There was an outdoor jogging path. All of them were *abbreviated* – enough to say they have them.

Contrast that with: The Casino? Huge, luxurious, and detailed – you could almost get lost in there. The Sports Bar? Had every game you would need! The arena for the shows? Took up 4-5 decks in the middle of the boat. The outdoor hot tubs and pools with surrounding bars and over-flowing buffets? Non-stop and fully stocked. Burgers. Pizza. Wings. High carb foods. Even when we docked in Cozumel, there were more bars, more restaurants – more shopping (In case I forgot, there was an abundance of shopping available on board as well.)

None of those were *abbreviated*.

We don't view working out as a vacation by itself. Is there a ship where the opposite is marketed to us? A ship dedicated to multiple levels of fitness with only an abbreviated bar, casino or shows. Does that exist?

Would that ship have portion control? Vast fermented foods? An international variety of fresh vegetables? Healthy grains from all parts of the world? That's not part of our vacation culture. Our subconscious wants to be rewarded with having access to decadent food & drinks around the clock. And here it was, laid out for us.

In my experiences inside your doctor's office, our vacation and comfort zone culture *manifests* inside a unique room – and not the examination room. Let's leave this cruise and let's take a walk inside the pharmaceutical drug closet.

CHAPTER 6

Healthcare & Emotional Wellness

METRICS. PSYCHOLOGY. PSYCHIATRY. PILLS

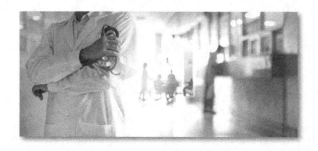

Fall 2010. Fairfax, Virginia

While wearing our finest professional attire, you and I will now visit the office of Doctor A. Smith: General Practitioner.

As per protocol, we initially check in at the front desk. The staff automatically knows that you and I are representatives of some corporate entity because we're the only ones dressed in suits in this waiting room (plus I visit this office frequently, they just haven't seen *you* before). This office is packed in here today, so with quick pleasantries, they just wave us along and we stroll into the back.

You and I walk towards the rear of the office and into the drug closet. It's a room – usually the size of a large bathroom – stacked with shelves of medication samples. Pharmaceutical companies ration out these free samples to doctor's offices so that patients can try them out before a doctor prescribes that specific medication.

So, close the door behind you and stand next to me inside this drug closet and let's observe. Take your time and scan what's stocked and available. Notice that none of it is exactly gathering dust.

- High Blood Pressure pills? Check. Middle shelf. Easy to find. From ACE inhibitors to Vasodilators. Dozens of companies make them.
- Diabetes Medications? Check. Don't just check the shelves in this closet. Look over here at this 'fridge. Tons of companies make these meds.
- Erectile Dysfunction? Check. Right here on your left. Not as many companies, but they're never in short supply.
- Sleep pills? Top shelf. They're supposed to be "put away" but I guess this whole closet is supposedly off limits. You and I are here to make sure this doctor has enough of a supply of samples from my company. Because as a nation, we're not just stressed about our health, we need major assistance sleeping.

We're inside of a space of healthcare that is rarely seen by anyone outside the industry, so let's talk for a quick second. How many of these medications are necessary because of our obesity issues as a nation? Some? All?

Whether fairly or unfairly, the international pharmaceutical industry is seen by many as villains within our community. It's not just that they have a reputation for being capitalist monsters, they are seen as intentionally *manipulating* the health of their consumers and the healthcare system.

I've been inside some corporate headquarters as an employee, and on interviews, in Thousand Oaks California, Chicago, and Research Triangle in North Carolina to name a few locations. Some of these companies' campuses are luxurious and modern enough to rival any resort in the Caribbean. Gorgeous, modern facilities. Corporate America, at its finest.

But come back from daydreaming about those corporate campuses and back into this doctor's drug closet. Let's walk back out into the hallway so we can speak with Dr. Smith.

We give her updates on our company's products and ask for her commitment to prescribe. But before we walk away, listen to her lament to her staff about how she could not get her patient in room 3 to *listen* to her about losing weight and being healthier. Hold on to her comments. We'll come back to them later.

Now let's stroll into the waiting room to see – us. All of us.

If you didn't notice it on your way in, notice it now. A lot of us are sick and in this waiting room with a litany of ailments. And to Dr Smith's point, we frequently do not want her advice *as much as* we want those pills in the drug closet. Our subconscious just wants to make itself happy with as little disturbance to its routines as possible.

My point is, just like we can't comprehensively blame the food, restaurant, or entertainment industries for being multi-billion-dollar entities, we can't wholly fault Big Pharma for *all of us* being in this waiting room (or walking onto that cruise ship). Supply and Demand? We're the ones demanding these pills *against* the direct advice of many doctors. And make no mistake, it has been my job to convince the doctors to prescribe more meds.

We're done in this office. We can walk back to the parking lot. We have 6 more offices to visit today. Hop in the passenger seat.

I'm driving.

The REDI Network creates a discussion platform for delicate topics.

Chapter 6 is **E**xamining how our Healthcare system struggles to handle our emotional wellness.

We'll close out this section of the book on **E**xamining the subconscious.

All our conversations around the subconscious versus various industries are still completely relevant in this chapter. But make no mistake, this book is just as much about impacting our healthcare system as much as it is about our individual fitness goals.

There are three ways in which our current healthcare system struggles with our collective Emotional Wellness:

1 – Seeing both emotional sides of the fitness equation.
2 – Mental Health versus Emotional Wellness (which is medical psychiatry versus emotional psychology).
3 – When progress is not measurable.

There are also two ways we can be more self-aware to assist our healthcare industry:

1 – Recognize our cultural stigmas.
2 – Pill Culture Mentality.

Our healthcare systems struggle to truly capture the emotional distress on both sides of the fitness equation. Side one of this equation: The motivation for some citizens to lose weight is not limited to "looking better" in the mirror to or "being healthier" on the scale, but to get rid of the emotional social stigma associated with being overweight.

The amount of physical health issues that directly result from our obesity crisis is compounded by the emotional stress many citizens feel daily with "feeling fat" in this country. The judgment overweight people feel from "healthy looking" individuals is steep, but maybe not *as* steep as the judgement felt from within themselves. The multiplying effect of emotional stress generated by self-hate leads to additional efforts by many individuals in seeking harmful dietary coping mechanisms to be detailed further in Chapter 12.

Upon hearing about the topic of this book in its embryonic stages, some of my colleagues in the psychology field wanted to ensure this endeavor would not lead to "fat shaming". Meaning any conversation around obesity is so frequently drenched with judgement as to what is supposed to "look good" to our society that it increases the stress levels of those deemed "unworthy" by their semantics. I fully agree with their sentiments and sensitivity. These topics are specifically limited to health implications: individual and system wide; Not to demonizing humans who are otherwise healthy but may not fit into the ideological society's square-peg hole of "beauty".

Side two of the fitness equation is what we examined in the last chapter: The emotional manipulation from numerous industries leading to our citizens having varied levels of addiction to highly accessible unhealthy foods.

All solutions must include ways to help with emotional stigmas/traumas of being overweight as well as decreasing hospitalizations by increasing self-awareness and overall fitness.

Right now, emotional wellness is one of the most nebulous aspects of our entire healthcare system. It's not nearly as organized or funded as our physical-healthcare system of doctor's offices & hospitals, pharmaceutical & insurance companies. As a result, our culture doesn't fully embrace it – mostly through not just knowing what it is.

Emotional Wellness versus Mental Health

Youth Football Coach

For 10 years I volunteered to coach youth football in suburban Maryland. A fellow coach & friend of mine suffers from occasional anxiety in addition to mild depression. He was prescribed medications from a crowded, assembly-line style psych office. He texted me some of the medications names and doses once prescribed for him and we went over the pros and cons, side-effects, what to expect etc.

Two Quick Questions for non-healthcare professionals:

- Was that a mental or an emotional situation?
- When you read the words: "psych office", did you picture a psychologist or a psychiatrist?

My friend/fellow coach got his meds and by and large, it helped. He received treatments from a psychiatrist's office, with little to no dialogue behind the reasons for each medication. But what he and I talked about is how a conversation (or many) with a psychologist could uncover childhood trauma which *is* still causing his PTSD-type anxiety today.

That's our case study. Today it is still unresolved and ongoing like many USA citizens.

With the assistance from the pharma industry, we can indeed attempt to medicate psychiatric issues. We haven't found a way to do the same for emotional issues – and by "the same" I mean treat the underlying issue – not just prescribe pills – on a large scale backed by corporate entities.

Back to our discussion on obesity and SAM. The nebulous nature of Emotional Wellness creates *confusion* (and occasional judgement) about addressing the psychological tie-ins to obesity.

And while we're not doing an A+ job treating Mental Health (like with my friend the youth football coach) we're at least attempting to treat disorders of the physical brain.

Let's make these next points clear:

1. Mental Health disorders stemming from irregular chemistry of the physical *brain* can be medicated within our healthcare systems using therapeutics prescribed with the field of psychiatry to bring balance to biochemical molecular levels. This directly helps us with schizophrenia, bi-polar disorders, substance abuse disorders, Alzheimer's as well as other neurological conditions.

2. Contrast that with *emotional wellness* stemming from childhood trauma, a bad break up, job and financial stress, an unexpected loved-one's death. Discussions within the field of psychology can bring clarity to the mind.

3. Our health care system, in terms of funding and research, isn't *as* focused on point #2. Much less our subconscious food and entertainment industry even though it directly affects this system. In fact, as we'll find out in Chapter 12, it is likely adding to the biochemistry of our obesity problems.

4. In summary: our medical field of psychiatry is much more structured and precise than our nebulous umbrella field of psychology leaving both fields grasping to find the right balance for our citizens.

When Progress is not measurable

Numbers. Facts. Measurements. We use these for our medical objectives, assessments, and treatment plans.

Even within the pages of this book, we need critical data points to illustrate and/or support specific ideas.

We can't always put our emotions on a chart to monitor progress. We have no numbers, no figures, no measurements. American society can't readily measure our emotional starting point and subsequent improvement. Since it's difficult to measure, this continues to blur the line between emotional wellness and mental health disorders (see: my youth football coach/friend).

(To be clear, search results did show that Medicaid does indeed pay for a ton of *mental health* disorder assistance. Commercial insurances can indeed assist with lowering the costs of psychologist-office counseling, but the disparities of the assistance provided to everyone are wide.)

Society Self-Awareness versus Healthcare

Comparable to the international cultural diet differences we discussed at the end of chapter 5, we also have a cultural dilemma with diagnosing and treating emotional health.

We do indeed have segments of our society that feel comfortable in discussing their *emotional* issues with professionals. Unfortunately, there are so many of us more concerned with the potential judgment of coworkers, friends, family, and of course, self. The stigma and fear of having conversations with a professional on our deeper emotional issues is even greater than the fear from fear we discussed in Chapter 1 – a cheek swab.

Pill culture and The Drug Closet

That story at the beginning of this chapter was directly from fourteen years of my two decades in Corporate America having been in the pharmaceutical industry. I've witnessed our "pill mentality" culture countless times in countless health care offices. I've spoken informally about this topic for years with physicians and nurses and hospital administrators.

The international pharmaceutical industry catches its share of ire from the public. I am not here to apologize for them.

However, it's not just that the industry itself wants to push medications at us via the prescriptions of doctors. Frequently, *patients want* the least number of disruptions to their daily comfort zones as possible. And taking a few pills is literally only *seconds* out of each day. As opposed to trying to form new habits to be healthy. That takes weeks. Months.

What did that lady say at that conference in Philadelphia? *"Honey, people just want to go home from work and watch their shows"*.

And that's what we have. The pills themselves are merely a super convenient way to keep the habits we enjoy. The responsibility for improving our healthcare outcomes goes both ways. Once we examine our subconscious emotional attachment to the landmines that various industries put forth, we'll be more self-aware. And that's where we draw the line.

We're done with our day of visiting doctors' offices. We're done with the **E**xplore section of the book as well. We **D**iscuss next. And I know the perfect spot. Let's hit the strip-club. We don't even have to change clothes; we can go dressed just like this.

SECTION 3

Discuss E.Q.

CHAPTER 7

Self-Awareness

HOW WE SABOTAGE OUR INDIVIDUAL FITNESS GOALS

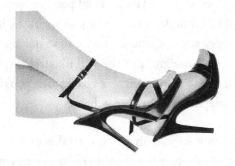

Spring & Summer 2009. Largo, Maryland.

Over the course of almost a 3-year span, there were an infinite number of individuals I trained at the now defunct Bally's Total Fitness in Capital Heights, Maryland. Only one of them is the singularly appropriate subject for this chapter. Her profession, more than most others, was contingent on her physical attributes. Without further ado, let's introduce one of my most favorite yet exasperating clients:

An exotic dancer.

Or stripper if you favor that expression because that is where she worked – at a strip club. I am confident no individual reading or hearing this chronicle would have even a picogram of disdain or contempt towards her occupation.

If in fact we are sincere regarding our ponderings on the ramifications of billion-dollar entertainment, pharmaceutical and restaurant companies' subliminal strategies while juxtaposing international cultural variances on diet and exercise, then unquestionably we can examine this factual woman with her tangible fitness challenges.

Excellent then.

This client of mine sought to lose 10 to 12 pounds to get into being in the "elite" shape she desired. Her body fat percentage was just over 26%. She wanted to get under 15%. If you saw her at the line in front of you at the grocery store, it would never cross your mind that this woman wanted to lose weight. But she still illustrates spectacularly just how difficult it is to achieve fitness goals when you're unwilling to trace your footsteps in order to break habits.

None of the words you read in the remainder of these next few paragraphs will truly capture her tenacity during our gym workouts. She had a run-through-brick-walls type of ferocity.

Free Weights? She attacked them like they had stolen something from her. Cardio? She would be so intense I would get frightened, for myself. Why frightened? Because I was in close proximity to this hydrogen bomb of a human being and the blast radius would certainly annihilate me. Core-work? I had to keep her pace slow so that she wouldn't hurt herself.

Companies like Bally's don't compensate trainers nearly as much as you would think, compared to what you pay as a consumer, so I was enthusiastic when she took her workouts to an additional level by hiring me to train her off site. Specifically, outside of brick-and-mortar

Bally's, we trained at a nearby community college track in Largo, Maryland. That's where this story catapults forward.

Witness her 100- and 200-meter sprints followed by intervals of walking slowly then walking quickly. High Intensity Interval Training. Her workouts were Olympic!

Yet, no matter how consistently her intensity stayed during our Largo track workouts, she erased that in her night-time diets when she went to work. At first, I thought it was for-lack-of-a-better-word "funny" when she would report back the next morning that she had her usual 2-3 alcoholic drinks, hot-dogs, or pizza (or both) which are all readily available at her club.

Then, through the days and weeks, it wasn't "funny" at all as she continued to work out hard and we continued to stress her diet more than her workouts.

Truth is, as I listened to her through the weeks, I became quite aware that she really liked those activities. And I don't mean the workouts at the gym or track. I mean the drinking, the clients, the atmosphere at the club. Our workouts: she marched through them without emotion. However, her descriptions of her previous night at the club always brought a sparkle to her persona.

Because of her enjoyment from the atmosphere of her work, she had clear, attainable goals and motives: Getting more attention and subsequent tip money in addition to being featured more on center stage through decreased body fat. She garners more money the more in-shape she is. Her goals were concretely realistic.

She even relayed to me before our very first workout that she observed that the women in her club making *serious* money were in better physical shape than she was.

Those incontrovertible goals and indubitable motivations were no match to get her to the point where she was going to give up what her SAM liked: Her down time. *Not just* her emotional attachment to the strip club culture.

As we mentioned in chapter 2, our conscious mind is commonly no match for SAM. Her beliefs and habits were not going to change despite her coherent and logical desires.

At various points in our lifetime of fitness journeys, we'll obtain an intense, elevated level of determination to get fit. For this particular performer, she was at that point right now. Consciously, she was ready to give blood, sweat and tears to run through figurative brick walls during our workouts. However, her subconscious was not willing to go further. It had no desire to manage her time before and after her shifts. It didn't desire planning because ultimately, it was gaining something *from* that whole vibe/scene at the club.

She was dismissive: *"yeah-yeah-sure-sure"* when it came to conversations about planning out her time *between* the track and the club. She agreed with the idea that she should eat healthily. She just couldn't follow through with the execution of managing her time to prepare those meals. SAM doesn't do well with time.

She believed she could throw herself into ferocious workouts while simultaneously not altering anything regarding the habits of her evening. Is this rational? Of course not.

And what was the result?

Did she have healthy, filling meals ready *before* she goes into her shift? No.

Did she take healthy snacks into the changing room to have available *during* her breaks? Not at all.

As her trainer, I couldn't jump out of the dressing room refrigerator to ensure she eats a beneficial meal during her break at 1:30am. (Mainly because I'm still at that restaurant/bar with the dim lights and the warm color schemes being manipulated to stay longer by the restaurant industry.)

Looking back on it. I wish I had done more to emphasize her time-planning. I wish I could have even gotten her out to the track and refused to train her on a day where she had refused to plan out her previous day. Or something. I feel like she was a petulant child, and I was a coddling parent.

I can't "measure emotions", but I "feel like" I could've done more.

What I wish I could have done is what we're **D**iscussing in this chapter. I wish I could ask her to re-trace her steps. How did she get to be 26%? How is it she was still at that level despite paying a trainer over the course of several weeks?

More importantly, I wish I could ask her to be more emotionally self-aware of what she truly enjoys about the *lifestyle* of her employment. I never went to see her perform. But I absolutely remember the way she gushed about the food, the drinks, and the clients with the exuberance of someone who loved all of it! She was emotionally attached to the exosphere of that performing stage. And her subconscious was unwilling to alter one thing.

You can't out-train your diet and you can't fool the desires of your subconscious – unless you directly **E**xamine it. Will-power cannot overcome beliefs and habits.

We worked out for weeks until… one day, a full week went by, and we didn't find the time to work out.

Then two weeks went by without a workout.

Then there weren't any more workouts in the gym or on the track. We didn't even get her final BF% measurements. I completely lost track of her.

The REDI Network creates a discussion platform for delicate topics.

The chapter is **D**iscussing how lack of Self-Awareness can sabotage even the most ardent of fitness goals.

Self-Awareness as part of Emotional Intelligence

In our last section of chapers, we explored the subconscious along with several entities that we're up against in the battle on obesity. As we stated many times in that section, we can't put all the burden of our health on those industries. The examination of our collective and individual responsibilities must be paramount.

Once we're self-aware of our individual emotional attachments, biases and preferences stemming from our subconscious, we're free to discuss with others without fear of being wrong or right. We can curb the relentless desires of the subconscious' attempts to "feel better" about itself. Self-awareness makes delicate discussions more malleable on the topics of romantic relationships, politics and media and of course, fitness and obesity.

The five parts of EQ:

1- Self-awareness: Being cognizant of your subconscious feelings and motives.

2- Self-regulation: Pausing and thinking of consequences before making impulsive decisions.

3- Motivation: Assessing the big-picture and seeing how actions can lead to long-term success.

4- Empathy: Becoming non-self-serving, excellent listeners with deep human compassion.

5- Social Skills: Not just the ability to work in teams, but to be excellent leaders that manage interpersonal relationships with aplomb.

For the purposes of this book, we will focus exclusively on the first two: Self-awareness & Self-regulation. And while this is a *collective* effort towards our overall levels of fitness, self-awareness and self-regulation begin with each of us as *individuals*. It starts with you.

We all need to have a clear grasp of our own feelings and *true motives* at any point in time. The question for the stripper would be, why wouldn't she want to plan healthy eating if she knew that could sabotage her goals?

Discuss those type of questions with yourself. (After all, it's called *self*-awareness for a reason.)

- How do you *really* feel about each of the individual aspects of losing weight?
- Specifically, the things you will not be able to do versus the things you will have to do that you may not enjoy (as my stripper client showed).
- What are your emotions about the journey?
- Is it something you will like (the idea of being healthy) or something you'll hate (the reality of giving up food you enjoy)?

When you're starting a new weight loss goal SAM's true motive will conflict with your objectives. And the industries we discussed in the earlier section will be what it wants to keep.

Still on the timeline of working as a personal trainer, these following questions came up all the time, and I know now they were derived from the subconscious ruminations of my clients:

- "I don't have to stop eating buffalo wings, do I?"
- "Is potato salad a vegetable or is 30g of sugar per serving too much in my orange juice? Because trying to find that stuff out takes *time*."
- "Can't I just take a pill?"
- How long will this take to reach those "goals"?

The Speed at which you achieve your goals =

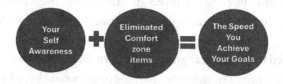

Your level of self-awareness + The number of items in your previous comfort zone habits you've identified as emotional attachments that can be reduced or eliminated.

Our subconscious is not adept at making new habits. But when we identify and discuss our emotional attachments to the landmines in our individual paths, we can reach our goals without battling our previous habits.

How to increase your Self-Awareness:

Trace your Footprints.

Self-awareness can help you re-set your habits. Step one is the surface level. Identify what habits got you here. Step two is to discuss your emotional attachment to those things.

How did I get here?

How did I get 20, 50, 100 pounds overweight?

How did my body-fat % exceed 30, 35, 40%?

How did my fitness level get to where I'm tired going up stairs and I stay tired most of the day?

Whatever your ideal weight or body fat% or fitness levels are: Can you trace exactly how you arrived at where you are? Sounds simple.

It's tougher than you think.

> "I was eating too much and not working out as much as I should."

Simple answer, right? It's the *"... as I should"* part that's tough. Because it lends to the thinking that if things were up to you, you'd do and eat the things you "should".

This is a **D**iscussion you have with your subconscious. Your conscious goals versus your subconscious desires. Lay it all out on the proverbial table.

The word Discussion: There's a line between **R**ealizing the conflicting motivations of our conscious and subconscious minds and discussing those motivations to be more self-aware. Discussions can be with professional counselors, loved ones, via meditation or just plain focus. That discussion is limited to any one method.

Let's go further on individual emotional attachments. There are three specific categories leading to subconscious self-awareness for our fitness journeys.

Categories X, Y, and Z

Your individual emotional attachments to X and Y and Z are all different.

It's not just that **X** (your list of the top 3-5 favorite unhealthy foods) is a different list than other people, but that you have your own unique emotional attachment as to why you consume them. (And that attachment is still separate from the food & restaurant industry setting us all up for consumption addiction.)

Y is your favorite activity that *isn't* conducive to your weight loss goal. Examples: lying in bed surfing social media or watching TV from the couch without moving for hours per week. Sitting at your desk at work is no longer a reason to be sedentary, there are too many companies and agencies that can create an active, ergonomic, standing workspace. The reasons you give for wanting to stay in a comfort zone of being sedentary are completely different reasons than other people.

Same with **Z** - the fitness activities you want to be doing. Going to the gym regularly, not periodically. Early morning running. Stretching before a workout. These are activities you need to increase but somehow you avoid. Discuss with your subconscious why these are difficult to maintain.

Now let's trace our footprints backwards.

That is, if you were at your *ideal* fitness level right now? What would be the steps you would take to arrive at your *current* fitness level?

That's right. How would you put on weight? What would you start eating? How would you lose muscle mass? How would you find ways to be more sedentary? We find ways to stay in our current situation. What are those ways?

Take as much time as you need to see your own footprints you made towards this path. Be as specific as possible, your self-awareness will help you when you're not reading this book or feeling super motivated. Your self-awareness will need to rescue you during days, hours, and moments where you'll reach for the XYZ comfort level you've had for years.

You're either going to decide to examine and then discuss your emotional attachment to the XYZ items that got you to your current weight, or maybe you'll decide:

> "I see XYZ, and I want to keep them. Because examining why I like those things and then giving them up might make me someone different. I don't want to lose who I am."

I have absolutely heard this sentiment above many times when I was a personal trainer. It was confusing to me initially, but quite a few amounts of people think they need to *be someone different* to drastically change their fitness/weight.

That's exactly the disconnect between your conscious fitness goals and what SAM fears when it hears those goals. Going back to the beginning of this book, it's the reason why people avoided a simple check swab: They may have to change their habits.

It's your *habits* that SAM has grown and vigorously works to maintain. It isn't merely about which diet or meal-plan, or gym or workout routine is the best for you. Of course, those things are important biologically. I, of all people, agree with that.

What can you understand about your emotional outlook on the whole task before you start "day 1" of your fitness journey?

It isn't just the food industry or television that can get in the way of our fitness goals. Our habits – make that *your* habits and beliefs - are exposed during numerous moments during the fitness journey.

Our habits and beliefs take time to change. **E**xploring those habits, those beliefs is a great initial step towards emotional intelligence. **D**iscussing *why* that emotional attachment *to* those habits and beliefs exists is a true full step towards self-awareness.

We mentioned at the beginning of this chapter how super-natural the stripper was in her workouts. Let's stay with that gym environment and **D**iscuss men in fitness.

CHAPTER 8

Self-Awareness

MEN IN THE FITNESS WORLD

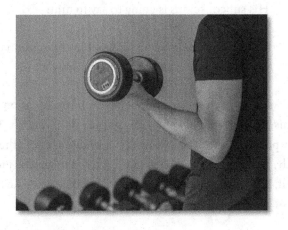

Winter 2008. Cleveland, Ohio.

Here comes Tom through the front doors. He hasn't set foot in this gym for a little over one year. He has never been go-to-the-gym type of guy. Usually, he walks or jogs a bit on the treadmills. Today, he is determined to start lifting weights.

He begins walking towards the free weights area in this crowded facility. He scans the available benches for his initial exercise today: The Bench Press. Finally, he spots an empty bench. Wouldn't you know it? The available bench is *right next to* some guy benching 315 pounds like celery.

Tom knows he's going to start with "just" loading a 25-pound weight on each side of the bar, which will bring the total weight of this chest exercise to 95lbs.

He hasn't even started loading the weights on the bar. But already Tom can feel that the *optics* of the 95 pounds on his bar versus the 315 being lifted by the guy next to him. Those optics will make him appear - well - weak. He is about to have a serious internal struggle with SAM. His subconscious is going to say to him:

> "I do not have enough security about my masculinity
> to feel comfortable lifting next to this guy."

Now if Tom were in this gym completely by himself - or on a bench-press in his house near Shaker Square - 95 pounds may not be ideal, but Tom may proceed because he won't feel the judgment of others. More accurately, if he were alone, he would better manage the judgement of himself. It's difficult to manage that inner voice when he perceives the eyes of everyone on him in this crowded gym.

Tom is having projections. His subconscious is projecting *its* judgement *into* the other people the gym: Those projections scream at him:

> "Everyone is noticing! The entire gym will pause and
> see me. And judge me."

No matter how secure we are, we all tend to overestimate how much other people notice us. Our own self-importance will make the weight of other people's eyes on us seem like blistering examination. And judgement.

Tom's projections continue:

> "The gap between what I'll be lifting and what he's
> already lifting will seem monumental."

Again, SAM is irrational. Everyone else in this gym is absolutely minding their own business. But you can't convince Tom of that, as he is actively seeking the eyes out of those around him to see how many of them might be looking his way. Anyone he makes fleeting eye contact with – according to his SAM – is gearing up to judge him.

His subconscious continues its assessment of the situation:

> "This other guy isn't just lifting 315 pounds easily;
> he'll start judging me when he sees me lifting 95
> measly pounds."

Here's what Tom does not know about that guy next to him lifting 315lbs. Ten months ago, that same guy walked into this very gym, sat down at the exact same bench press that Tom is pausing in front of now and that guy could only bench-press 65 pounds. He put a 10-pound weight on each side of the 45-pound metal bar. And he *struggled* to lift that amount.

If Tom knew that, if he knew that the guy lifting 315 was at one point *working his way up to* the 95 that Tom can already lift now? Tom might be inspired. Tom's insecurities might be soothed.

But Tom has no access to that information. And SAM is only seeing what's in front of it. With its all-knowing memory, it's protecting itself from more harm, in the form of ridicule that it's already experienced earlier in childhood that had nothing to do with lifting weights but affects his view of his own masculinity.

And since SAM doesn't understand time, it will compile *that* experience with this potential experience in the very real and current present. Again, Tom hasn't even started loading the weights on the bar yet there is *no way* SAM is exposing itself - in this gym today - to more potential embarrassment.

Consciously, Tom had all the willpower in the world before he came to the gym - in terms of the benefits of lifting weights. He doesn't merely want to get stronger. Tom consciously knows building lean muscle mass will help burn calories even when he's not at the gym. He is also consciously aware that it will take time to build the frame and strength that he wants.

All this assessment and subconscious reflections that took you a few moments to read in the previous pages took Tom's subconscious less than ten seconds to process while standing in front of that empty bench. And what transpired? His willpower was no match for SAM. It wasn't a fair fight and didn't last one round. SAM knocked out Tom's conscious willpower in one punch and got him the heck out of that weightlifting area of the gym.

As we can see, Tom has now meandered in the treadmills area. A short while later, Tom's subconscious will remind its passenger that he *never enjoyed going to the gym in the first place.* His subconscious will put Tom in the passenger seat and drive them both back to his house.

Go back to the guy lifting 315. He was a complete stranger. Do you think Tom would benefit if next time he brought his own friends with him to the gym?

Well, if those friends load on more weight than Tom when it's their turn - and even worse - take off those weights when it's *Tom's time to lift* 95lbs? Tom will still feel internally intimidated and inferior, so he'll probably avoid that situation, even though they're his friends.

While the exotic dancer was a real person, there are more broad examples I've witnessed as a trainer in a major health club and as a Pilates instructor. Most of the examples have little to do with the actual workouts inside those facilities. It's the general insecurities many males feel towards wanting to come to the gym or studio.

While he is a fictitious character, "Tom" is directly based on numerous male colleagues, friends, and family members of mine. Many of them share these exact sentiments as to why they won't venture to the gym or attend a group class. They know the benefits of health. Unfortunately, they're uncomfortable. (Read: intimidated) by the gym environment.

Their concerns are: Not lifting as much or more weights or being as in shape *as other men* will make them feel like less of a man. It's a cultural phenomenon: many guys feel like they need to *already* be physically strong – and starting a journey to be stronger means just that – starting. And that starting point of current physical "weakness" is too emotionally taxing for so many males.

Is this rational? No.

But if you've felt like less of a man in any other capacity or been told by someone that you're less of a man. Or been bullied. Teased. Then your subconscious - who only sees things in the present - will see this potential lifting experience, irrationally. It will compile all the other "less of a man" instances and make sure *that feeling* doesn't come up by *avoiding the situation*.

And it works both ways: The other side of the exact same coin.

Some men do indeed "feel better about themselves" when they are working out with 315 on the bench press. Not just physical strength.

They feel more confident in social circles when they get noticed as someone who *"clearly works out"*.

Just like it shouldn't lead towards feelings of insecurity when men can only lift 95lbs; It shouldn't lead towards feelings of superiority when a male can lift 315. Yet both exist.

And inexorably, if Tom had a home gym and a few months and got up to 315 pounds, unless he was self-aware enough to recognize and flesh out the origins of his insecurities, he will absolutely judge the next "95-pound lifter" who risks lifting next to him. Fundamentally, Tom projected what he would feel if he *could* lift 315 pounds towards himself.

Insecurity without it. Arrogance with it. It's the same coin.

Tom's subconscious drove him back home safely. He didn't lift one weight today. We thank him for his example.

The REDI Network creates a discussion platform for delicate topics.

This chapter is here to Discuss the different Self-Awareness issues Men face in our overall fitness culture.

Emotional intelligence through self-awareness provides a full cup of self-esteem that is neither diminished nor enhanced by the amount of weight lifted on a bench.

But you say: *"well how does that happen"*? How does one get to the point of that level of self-awareness?

Because it sure sounds great to say "don't be intimidates by":

- those lifting more weights than you.

- or driving a "better" car than you.
- or making more money than you.
- or living in a bigger house than you.

Sounds great to say don't become cocky or arrogant if you have garnered the "impressive" bench press, car, house, or job.

These items have traditionally been societal hallmarks derived from many previous generations, of how a man can "define" his maleness. Be physically strong. Acquire a stylish automobile. Garner a robust job title accompanied by the requisite strapping salary. Own a home with curb appeal. Have an attractive partner whom other men would deem "attractive".

Society sees those things on the surface and interprets that this male is living up to "the standards" and even surpassing those standards. That approval lends to the male SAM – the male ego - being able to "feel better" about itself. However, the insecurities and lack-of-self-esteem that needed to be "boosted" by a better job, a bigger house, a trendy car or a higher bench-press, may very well be still present despite acquiring these items. Thus, the relentless pursuit continues.

Self-awareness, joined by self-regulation via discussions with a loved one, therapist or other healthcare professionals can diagnose the *gap* between your self-esteem, and what gets filled from a house, job, car, bench-press. That gap is the reason you're comparing yourself in the first place.

Not to be forgotten. A lot of this dynamic about working out in a public place does indeed fall on the culture of the institution itself. There are entire marketing campaigns directly aimed at getting folks into facilities that don't have a judgment mentality.

But that's the point. Your subconscious may be the target of advertising executives sitting in a meeting room at Planet Fitness headquarters saying: *"I bet a lot of people are intimidated by their projections about "in-shape" people. How can we cash in on that?"*

It's crafty and effective marketing, but it's not helping tons of people whose subconscious' needs remain unresolved as they go for another round of pizza while agreeing to sign on at (Mars, Saturn, Neptune & Jupiter) Fitness gym.

Back to men at the gym

By no means are we saying women don't face societal pressure to look fit, feminine or be financially fabulous, etc. There are tons of women sabotaging their fitness goals by unfairly comparing themselves to their peers or images on social media. In my experiences in the fitness world, there are more women than men willing to face those fears and dive into their own emotional, self-awareness journeys which results in them showing up at a fitness facility. Unfortunately, there are too many men still struggling with being emotionally and physically vulnerable.

Vulnerability isn't limited to appearing weak or feeble for men in the gym. It's fear of a judgement-filled concept from our Neanderthal-era culture.

In my time in healthcare and fitness industries, men are more likely than women to become arrogant once gaining the dense, lean muscle mass physique which society has told us equates to masculinity. That arrogance, wafting over from that guy lifting 315 pounds is something insecure men lifting 95 pounds can project (imaginary) or sense (real) and feel intimidated by their *lack* of that male-defining trait. It leads to the vicious cycle we saw with Tom.

Too many men won't get started with their fitness gyms because consciously they're comparing their male strength to the other males in the gym. However, their subconscious is comparing feeling insecure *now* to feeling insecure in non-linear timeline of past childhood trauma.

In addition, for generations, many of our current definitions of masculinity were wrapped up in being not just physically strong but being emotionally tough. The "Boys don't cry" type of ideology.

I can't tell you how happy I am that a lot of this mentality has changed in my lifetime. But there are still many of my male friends and family members who judge themselves like "Tom".

Group Classes

In the fitness world, self-judgment is not just prevalent in the gym. It's not merely confined to the testosterone-laden bench press. America also experiences this in the group class setting.

While the example of an aerobics class is the most obvious instance, the expanding yoga and Pilates worlds still see far more women than men. Through 7 years of being an instructor, on average I see about a 75-25 ratio in my classes and the same ratio when I attend other instructor's classes for my own fitness.

Fear of being judged in a group class could be remarkably similar to being petrified at a middle school dance.

Is that Rational? Of course not. But if SAM can avoid the situation, it will.

It's not just because of lack of strength or being in shape. Self-judgment wouldn't allow several of my male friends, coworkers, and family members to engage in poses or positions that - in their minds - look feminine.

Again, it's Neanderthal mindset:

> "I'm not sure I'm masculine enough to overcome my self-judgment in these classes, so I'll just avoid or belittle those type of events".

We men are absolutely allowed to ask for a spot (another person to assist slightly) as we're about to bench-press 315 lbs. That's a fully masculine activity.

No problem.

Stretching in a "compromising" position in a yoga class? Or even tougher: asking for an emotional "spot" as we grapple with how to Discuss a potential disconnect with our subconscious? For too long those have been viewed as feminine activities.

Problem.

Even further down the Neanderthal-era brain level thinking: Not only are those activities frequently viewed as *not masculine,* but in groups of just males, they can be ridiculed. And it's been this way for decades.

Males discussing emotions? Traditionally, in a stereotypical chauvinistic 1950s setting, the only time males talk about emotions are to describe them as a popular female topic of conversation.

There is good news: The group class gender dynamic is slowly changing. More men are feeling comfortable in a group-fitness class setting. More men are feeling comfortable Discussing their emotions. The trend is growing - slowly.

There is bad news: Our USA obesity rates are not going up *slowly.* They are increasing steadily – by some metrics, rapidly.

Our culture's masculinity standards do not lend themselves to discussing "fears and insecurities" among peers, much less in a psychologist's office. This book encourages both. If there is an opportunity for open discussions on emotions – do it.

Guys like Tom in our society have been so common throughout my years in healthcare and fitness that *this is the first group* I thought about from chapter 1 while driving back from that conference in Philadelphia.

Remember: Patient's relatives feared getting that cheek swab to test for a rare disease. Low self-esteem males like "Tom" not only have to face their fears of self-judgment at the gym, but they also lack the self-awareness to confront the underlying, non-time-dependent, childhood trauma, pressure and/or neglect that generated the self-judgment in the first place.

Additional parallels to that conference in Philly:

The existing resources which could relieve self-judgement, thus increasing individual self-awareness for this group of guys are currently not visible to them and thus, underutilized. (Staggering resources met with thunderous fear.) Gyms, fitness classes, meditation practices and other wellness professionals and facilities are available yet unable to assist these males. Bars, cigar lounges, restaurants with ambiance and the entertainment of social and mainstream media will continue to babysit their subconscious' emotions.

Tom would rather be at the bar (right across from me) or cigar lounge where he consciously feels immediately accepted as soon as he has a seat. In those safe places, his subconscious doesn't have any reminders of past childhood trauma. As opposed to that bench at the gym starting at 95 pounds, where he must work out for *months* - at the minimum – to feel better about himself.

As this group ages and continues to lack self-awareness, their increased chances of poor health will continue to populate the waiting rooms of our Dr. Smith. They will also increase the costs for our state-funded, government insurances, making this group an issue for all of us.

Once again, we thank "Tom" while witnessing him struggle emotionally in the gym today. I mentioned that "Men in Fitness" was the first group of people I thought about on that ride from Philly to DC. Next, my mind went to a female friend of mine struggling with her obesity for many years. Her story can help us all with the topic of self-regulation.

CHAPTER 9

Self-Regulation

WORK WITH YOUR EMOTIONS, NOT AGAINST THEM

August 2019. Lake Arbor Maryland.

A dear friend of mine has been attempting to lose 100-125 pounds for almost two decades of her life. In previous years, to no avail, she and I endeavored to set up a length of time for her to lose weight. We also attempted to set up an overlapping time frame for me to work on my entrepreneur endeavors (and potentially get in elite shape myself). We've been trying to set up all this seemingly forever.

This time in August 2019, at one of our favorite Prince George's County venues, with one of our other friends joining us, we finally constructed a 54-week time frame ending with the Labor Day weekend 2020 to attain our independent goals. Along the way, we'd be inspiring and supportive to each other.

During this same outing, we also came up with our reward *after* we accomplished our goals: A chartered boat with the rest of our circle of former coworkers and current friends in the Mediterranean Sea. We had the plan fully formulated: We'll hit a few islands: Ibiza, Santorini, Cyprus, we'll generate further details of the reward as we get closer to our goals.

But at the time, while we were still in the planning phase, we thought - before we each began our journeys, we'd take one final opportunity to go all out. That is, one last final Pig Out Meal Extravaganza. So, at this local restaurant, we dove into their menu of fantastic saliva-inducing, greasy, creamy, crunchy food selections. (We didn't stay there long after we ate, that restaurant had far too many windows.) We called/texted a few others and got them involved in this "farewell to decadence" occasion. We went barhopping to two more of our favorite nearby watering-holes immediately after our pig out, to add even more calories to the day.

Sounds like fun times.

Emotionally what were we *really* doing?

The message we're really conveying to SAM is: These are activities that we like: Eat decadent food at our favorite restaurants, matriculate to our favorite bars. Additionally, we're also imparting that the task we're about to embark upon is one where we won't be able to do things we like. We're going to sacrifice "fun times" for a jail-like-sentence for a full year. And then, somehow, we'll emerge on the other side of the jail sentence laughing about it on a Mediterranean island.

How long did it last? How far into the timeframe did we make it? Take a guess.

Just about as long as any New Year Resolution commitment to losing weight: A few weeks to a few months.

However, there was a slight difference in our results: I didn't get as far as I *wanted* in that time frame, but I did get a lot done.

Is that because I had more *Willpower*? More Discipline? Am I a better person?

No, it's because I wasn't sacrificing as much. Authoring books and starting a business requires focus and attention, yes. Good days and slow days, yes. But those are things (especially writing and researching) that I naturally enjoy doing. For me, SAM isn't compromised. I'm not making it do things it doesn't like. Those things are all working *with* my emotions.

Contrast that with my friend. Think about SAM driving her car. By setting a reward before and after, she's *not only* saying directly to SAM:

- You can't go to bars.
- You can't eat what you like.
- You must readjust your entire comfort-zone time frames of your daily

She's also re-emphasizing to her SAM that this is a huge sacrifice. A long jail sentence at a maximum-security facility. Ironically, it's almost the equivalent behavior people do before they *literally* go to jail: Live it up big and we'll see you when you get out.

SAM is *not* going to just drive itself to the local prison and check itself in for an extended stay. In fact, it's probably laughing at the whole idea on "Day One of The New Healthy Routine to Lose Weight and Cruise to Cyprus", also known to SAM as: The Jail Sentence.

Here is one more reminder: SAM doesn't understand linear time.

> "Sacrifice for a year?
>
> Jail for a year? A what? A beer?"

No, a year.

> "Well, what the heck is that? You want me to drive where for what? No thanks."

In addition, she is asking SAM to spend more time going to the store to acquire fresh foods (that spoil more rapidly, even in the fridge) and make her schedule work to hit the gym or step-class or go walking etc.

SAM wants to order delicious pizza and wings from an app while sitting at home watching TV.

Another reminder, this is not a fair fight as SAM is more powerful of an operating system for our emotions. After a week or two, a highly aggravated SAM will be more than annoyed at her repeated yet futile attempts to consciously take the wheel and drive where *she* wants to go.

The REDI Network creates a discussion platform for delicate topics.

Chapter 9 is here to **D**iscuss how our subconscious can sabotage our fitness goals through a lack of Self-Regulation

---

From our previous chapter on Men in Fitness, we see how self-awareness can lead to identifying the issues we may face on our fitness journeys, but what about the next step in the process? But how do we regulate ourselves even once we have done a true exploration of the subconscious?

What's the tangible plan? Week by week. Day by day. Hour by hour. How do we change our habits?

"The subconscious mind is a habit mind and the most important thing about a habit mind is that you don't want it to change very quickly because otherwise habits fall apart. So, it is resistant to change. It's not as easy to change as the creative mind". (Lipton, n.d.)

From our conversation on Emotional Intelligence comes: Self-regulation.

This is the ability to not make impulsive decisions. Self-regulation tactics monitor old habits or create new ones. It alerts us to deviations from diets and avoidance of day-by-day temptations that arise *after* that initial emotion of determination fades.

This chapter will discuss three different methods for creating new habits using various levels of rewards. All three of these rewards systems are dependent on the individual being self-aware first!

Rewards can be like the proverbial carrot in front of the horse to keep it moving along. You can absolutely pick one that seems better for you.

Reward Theory 1:

Grit
Will power and hard work.

In this theory, you don't need to reward yourself for working hard or doing well. The reward is accomplishing your goal. The stripper client illustrates this method.

This is the Angela Duckworth "grit" mentality. This theory has been documented and chronicled for getting humans in a variety of learning situations to develop new habits and get results.

And it works for so many people. If this is something that can work for you in your fitness journey? I'm all for it! Have at it. Or maybe it can work for a few weeks or months at a time.

Let's examine further.

"Research shows grittier people are happier. We should note, however, that it is a rewarding kind of accomplishment happiness, not 'fun' happiness. And we should not mistake that it is not always fun to work hard." (Duckworth, n.d.)

A professor at the University of Pennsylvania, she focuses mostly on the learning environment in schools and states that:

ACHEIVEMENT = TALENT times EFFORT

Can we apply this as well to losing weight?

Take whatever interests you have in the weight loss world that you enjoy. (Walking, cycling, step classes etc.) and multiply that by the EFFORT to avoid the specific foods you identify that are blocking you from being fit.

Grit is as straightforward as that. The only issue for me is that SAM would have to be 100% in agreement with everything we're about to do. Each of us would have to love every aspect of the fitness journey, from new workouts to new diets to rearranging our daily schedules.

In summary, in short bursts, Grit is very doable.

Self-Regulation Reward theory 2:

See the activities as something you enjoy.

July 2020. I was about halfway through my writing of the first book on Narcissism, Politics and Media: Triangle Games. A buddy of mine called and I gave him an update on my progress. He wanted to commend me on how "disciplined" I was on writing the book. He said:

"*Man, you stay so focused on these books, how do you do it, what's your secret?*"

He couldn't see me over the phone, but his question had me putting my shoulders up near my ears as I shrugged. I tried to explain that... well... I just like writing. And I like doing research for writing. I had no real explanation for him, and I had never given any thought about the concept of being "disciplined". For me, it's difficult to stop writing/researching (unless someone wants me to meet them at the bar).

I did mention to him that no one ever tells me how "*disciplined*" I was for being at happy hour the other day. Or asks "*what's my secret*" on how and when to order another round of drinks for the table. No one says: "*Jay you stay so focused on when to order the next round man. How did you know it was time for that?*"

My subconscious doesn't view writing books, working out or being at happy hour as a jail sentence, therefore I don't need to reward it for a productive week of writing (or happy hour). Just doing either of those are rewards in of themselves. I don't need to re-wire my brain to do those things.

But imagine if I had rewarded myself because I had stayed "disciplined" writing that book. Imagine if a good week of writing was followed by Friday night rewards of wings, TV, and social media. In that instance, I'm signaling to my subconscious that Monday through Friday was a grind, a jail sentence, something I needed to reward myself for surviving.

If you view the *journey* towards your goal as reward itself, SAM doesn't feel the need to reward itself. The more you tell yourself you like it. The more SAM will believe it loves it. You consciously like it. SAM loves it.

This helps especially when your subconscious wants to reward itself with items that go against your fitness goals: those scrumptious, calorie-heavy, non-nutritious food!

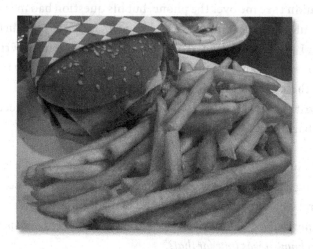

You can *never* have a reward system which goes *against* what you're trying to accomplish. You can't reward yourself for losing ten pounds by going out to binge on pancakes, syrup, and bacon.

My dear friend from the beginning of this chapter once told me all about the actor and fitness enthusiast Dwayne "The Rock" Johnson and his meal-cheat-days as to how not everyone has to eat healthily *all the time*. My response goes with the reward systems we're discussing in this chapter:

> "That's great, he's already in shape, he's not trying to lose 100 pounds and he's super strict with his diet and workouts on the days when he's not doing a Cheat Day. Plus, he has trainers and agents and other people to keep him on track because his career depends on him marketing an image of a fitness professional. If that fits your situation 100%? Then by all means, enjoy your pancakes."

I wouldn't "reward" myself for a productive week of writing by deleting the last five pages of what I wrote. Right?

That would be a double dose of damage to my long-term and short-term goals. Short term is obvious: I have less pages to show for this week. Long-term, this theory #2 is that rewarding myself with anything makes my subconscious view this past week as a jail sentence it had to survive.

You can still:

- Identify items that keep you from getting to your goals then,
- Evaluate your emotional attachment to those items (satisfying SAM) then,
- Not have to reward yourself when you reach your daily, weekly, or monthly goals.

If you go to the gym and you're labeling this as your daily workout *and you don't like working out*, you're more likely to seek a reward of FOOD that goes against your fitness goals.

"You can will yourself to go to the gym if you don't feel like it for a few days. But unless the gym ends up feeling good in some way, you will eventually lose motivation, run out of willpower and stop going. You can will yourself to stop drinking for a day or a week, but unless you feel the reward of not drinking, then you will eventually go back to it. Any emotionally healthy approach to self-discipline must work with your emotions, rather than against them." (Manson, n.d.)

If you are preparing a salad and your mind is labeling this as a diet and *you don't like the idea of giving up pasta and wings* then again, SAM is protesting giving up what it likes and is gearing up to make you hate that salad!

Key words in that quote *"unless you feel the reward."* Not that you reward yourself with any other item, but that the gym or quitting drinking is the reward itself.

For this Self-Regulation theory #2: setting up a rewards system means what you're going to attempt is something you don't really want to do. You could potentially be setting up your mind to reject (either over time or very quickly) the idea that you're going to punish it to achieve your fitness goals.

Just even thinking about the physical activities as fun or enjoyable and the process of healthy eating as enjoyable may be enough to re-wire SAM into habits that it won't need to protest.

"Engaging in a physical activity seems to trigger the search for reward when individuals perceive it as exercise but not when they perceive it as fun. We suggest that framing exercise as fun reduces individuals' tendency to indulge because it diverts their attention away from the effort required by the physical activity." (Werle, 2014)

That article illustrates one of the biggest subconscious' ways of sabotaging our fitness goals: *Our perception of our fitness journey before we even get started.*

Here is how you can re-wire the subconscious: Use the power that SAM has for your goals, not against your goals. When you say you like it, when you practice seeing the whole ordeal as fun, SAM will amplify it and say it loves it. SAM is a much more powerful super-computer than our 1960s IBM Apollo-mission CPU.

So again, if you don't fully enjoy those workouts or diets, reframe them as fun and enjoyable.

(Rewards) "teaches us that we'd do this activity only if a reward is offered. A reward provides extrinsic motivation, which tells us that we don't feel intrinsic motivation. We're not practicing guitar because we want to practice guitar but because we promised ourselves a beer every time we practice." (Rubin)

Self-Regulation Theory Three

Limited Reward system
Momentum

May 2020. The headaches were crippling, and it was now almost two weeks straight.

As with many people during the 2020 pandemic shutdown, I struggled with my fitness in the days and weeks of that COVID19 spring quarantine.

When the pandemic first hit in mid-March. Many businesses were closed, and it still wasn't nice enough weather outside to hit the track. But because of the momentum I had going from my workouts in January and February, initially in March & April I was still going strong, working out in my house 1-3 times a day.

Then in early May, I got those headaches, and they weren't from Covid19. They came from staring into this bright computer screen all day working on what would eventually turn into what you're reading right now. It ended up being three weeks of crushing headaches and throbbing neckaches.

I formed a new habit: not working out.

All I could do for most of those two weeks was lie in the dark to try and relieve my headaches. (I got new contact lenses and readjusted my screen, it was fine.)

Months later, it was difficult for me (someone who enjoys working out) to get going again with in-house workouts. I'd call it momentum. SAM is the one that needs time to build and trust any new routines.

It was well into the fall that I got back to my in-house routines. I still wasn't going to the gym to lift or the Hot Yoga Studio because the novel coronavirus never reached levels where I felt comfortable in those environments.

But the point is, I still needed a reward system to get me going again. Just to build momentum. I fully recognize that making a huge deal of rewards creates a line of thinking within SAM that working out in the basement in punishment and not "enjoyable".

I set up rewards for the end of each week that if I reached my fitness goal for week one, I'd treat myself with some streaming movie.

Week two, I had to come up with a different reward (and not plan it two weeks in advance, create it that Monday, the week of) which ended up being yardwork because the weather cooperated to be sunny and high 60s.

I understood that if I just viewed the in-house workouts as *enjoyable,* I wouldn't need any reward. No movies, no yardwork, just a successful week of writing and basement workouts.

But I just needed to get going after months of my *new habit* which had been formed from May until October: Nothing, Nada, Zip (well, an occasional journey to the track when it wasn't an inferno outside during summer.)

But once I got going with just two weeks of October/November basement workouts, I didn't need any more rewards. The blood-rush of workouts made it enjoyable on its own. (By the way, all I have in the in-house is a yoga mat and my own body weight. A pull up bar. No other equipment.)

The point is: We can compare this whole "in-house workouts" and momentum to tons of other people who haven't been working out on a regular basis and therefore, don't have any momentum going towards their goals.

I want to make this clear. There is no one way to do this for every individual, but there are not limitless options on tackling your fitness journey either.

1. Identify the handful of items that get in your way of your fitness goals. It's not a lot.
2. Identify an underlying emotional attachment to each item. If you feel like you can't, no problem, we'll work on that in an upcoming chapter on counseling.
3. Set up your plan. Whatever diet you like, whatever workouts you enjoy, and how you will manage your time.
4. Next: exactly what we're discussing right now. Can you just use willpower to create new habits? Can you see your *new lifestyle* as enjoyable and not a jail sentence? Do you need short-term rewards or long-term rewards or no rewards at all?

Again, once I got going. I didn't need rewards for weeks 3, 4 etc. I'm fully aware that the longer I need a reward, the more I might be seeing the workouts as not enjoyable and the more prone I'll be towards abandoning my goals.

Speaking of goals.

Even how you *set your personal goals* is a message to your subconscious.

If your goal is to lose fifty pounds: Sure, it's *great* once you start to consistently see weight loss: But the problem is *getting it going* and even saying "*I want to lose 50 pounds*" can be a message to your subconscious of a jail sentence.

Seeing the weight loss journey as a new lifestyle that is fun and enjoyable can be "*I can't wait to enjoy my new healthy lifestyle.*"

That last sentiment has more of a long-lasing fun message to SAM. We're about to do something FUN (and hey, if we happen to lose 50 pounds and look and feel wonderful, then we're not mad at that).

Before you get momentum, without the proper framing, all we can see is what we'll have to sacrifice. With the proper framing, we'll see the FUN we're about to have with a new style of living.

I'll start Monday:

My week is basically:
*Monday
*Monday #2
*Monday #3
*Monday #4
*Friday
*Saturday
*Pre-Monday

New Year's Day isn't the only time on the calendar where we try and start a new fitness routine. More than one of us has decided "I'll start Monday" when Monday is still a few days off and separated from us by a weekend emotional barrier.

We'll get ourselves in the "right frame of mind" to start again – a jail sentence of diets, workouts, and sacrifice. So, if today is Wednesday or Thursday, Monday seems far enough away that we'll be able to either sum up the courage to start or, magically it will stay Saturday or Sunday forever and we won't even have to do any new diet come Monday.

I could give you a pep-talk about starting today and looking at the list of four things a couple of pages ago that could get you going, but I'll just ask: why *do* you view it as something you want to put off?

"I'll start Monday" is of course, procrastination. We all procrastinate on doing things we really do want to do. But why?

- What does your subconscious enjoy while you are procrastinating?
- Are those procrastination activities a reward you're giving yourself?
- Why are those activities *more important* than the things that you say you want to achieve? Or are they?

If those questions are not something you can figure out in a day or so? We have an entire chapter on counseling and other methods coming right up. But any system, and self-awareness and subsequent self-regulation is better than going into a workout/diet plan *without* analyzing your subconscious emotional attachment to potential barriers to along your journey.

"Procrastination comes from some type of fear. If you are not consciously aware of such fears it's because they are, for the most part, subconscious fears. Those fears stop you from "physically" taking actions to move forward in life, and in order to stop you physically, your subconscious uses procrastination. This is the reason why most people who procrastinate have no clue or can't rationally explain why they do." (Nuccio)

Before we close this section, let's go back to that drive from Philly to open a chapter on getting started on this voyage. Vulnerability and the subsequent benefits of professional counseling are paramount on that journey.

CHAPTER 10

Discussing EQ isn't easy

VULNERABILITY + STIGMAS OF PROFESSIONAL COUNSELING.

October 2019. Philadelphia, Pennsylvania.

More specifically, the parking lot leaving that hotel, walking towards the car. There is always a first step on any journey, and this is it. The profound puzzlement I had over the patients' families who wouldn't take a simple check swab started before I even got to my car, much less behind the wheel.

It's understandable they had that fear because it's a *serious* disease. But was their attachment to that fear *that strong*? I couldn't wrap my brain around it, especially with all those outstanding resources willing to help.

Our individual journeys in the fitness world also can start with self-evaluation leading to self-awareness. Where does it start for you?

- Childhood struggles from a controlling or non-emotional parent.
- A bad romance or friendship separation?
- A tense job situation?
- Death of a loved one?

It can be tough to figure it out on your own. And even if you think you have a good handle on each item that could be emotionally standing in the way of you reaching your goals, how can you be sure that what you think is truly the answer?

There's a third person that can help you and your subconscious get on the same page so that you can be the one driving this vehicle.

Your Professional Counselor.

The REDI Network creates a discussion platform for delicate topics.

Chapter 10 is here to Discuss the difficulties of Vulnerability and the stigmas of professional counseling.

Every individual not only has different items that they're attached to that keep them from reaching their fitness goals, but different reasons for being attached.

Your reasons for not wanting to put down butter-pecan ice cream is vastly different than mine. But we can both have a conversation with a counselor starting with just that question:

"I can't figure out why my attachment to XYZ is so strong."

That's step one.

You could work on that question with family/friends and hopefully that could help. But working on it with a trained professional can help with the deeper issues.

But for many people who have never tried it or have only dabbled in the world of emotional therapy it leads to *more* issues:

- I don't want to be vulnerable.
- How would I even start to talk about this stuff?
- How do I find a good one?

"I don't want to be vulnerable."

It's Ironic. Our subconscious mind can make movies seem real, keep us craving foods that we know aren't good for us, entertain us by scrolling through a 2-by-5-inch screen for hours. But when asked to be potentially vulnerable to figure out why we do all these things? We'll pass.

Make no mistake, being emotionally vulnerable is not easy. And that's the point. We can get assistance for it in the same way we could get assistance via a personal trainer in a gym.

And being vulnerable is one of the first and largest steps towards overall emotional intelligence. Being vulnerable is tough in any situation. Many of the world's creatures who find themselves "vulnerable" find themselves quickly eaten by other species higher up the food chain. Vulnerable, by nature can be seen as fragile, weak, feeble. We admire the traits of being strong, commanding and being feared.

> "Opening up and talking to some stranger about what might be in my subconscious?"

That sounds scary for tons of people who may *not* want to open up and investigate. It may not be your childhood. It may not be a traumatic event from teenager years or early adulthood. It may be something that the supercomputer SAM is holding onto that you have completely forgotten about it.

Here's how it can work in real time conversation.

I opened-up a bit when I talked about my inner-child feeling "all grown up" when I sit at a bar and have a drink. A deeper dive with a therapist would be:

- "Why do you need to feel grown up?"
- What makes you *feel* better when you're eating food and having drinks made at a bar?
- Is it all about the alcohol itself? Is it about being served? Is it about socialization around other people?

It just gets you to think of what's behind the attachment. Sometimes you solve it during the session, sometimes it's homework for you to think about later.

> "What if I open up and someone doesn't understand me and then judges me based off that misunderstanding? I could be telling them about the issues that I think have led to my actions but because I'm not sure then they might fill in the gaps and mis-read me?"

The fear of being vulnerable is that we'll open ourselves to judgement. It's tough to *trust* that some person won't use this information against us. And we worry that the judgment we'll get from other people *will be worse* than the judgement we already give ourselves. Our subconscious holds us hostage with this information all the time and it's tough to separate the judgement we have of ourselves from the potential judgement we'll get from others. It seems so risky! We would be *destroyed* if others judged us. So, we'll just continue to keep it to ourselves for now, thanks for asking though.

You say where do I start?

A good counselor will start with just getting to know you. He or she will have their own techniques for that first session.

Thoughts you can have on your mind include: Your family life growing up. Your relationship with whoever raised you. Any person you wished had shown you more love while growing up. Any relationship or friendship patterns that you've seen, been told of, or now realize in hindsight. Physical places or emotional spaces in life where you visit that potentially you feel uncomfortable about. Social relationships that you have that have been fractured or are contentious.

Also, more of the things we've gone over in earlier chapters: Your fitness goals versus your comfort zone. Because the possibility of finding out what attaches you to your comfort zone activities could lead towards other insights within your life to discuss.

You're reading this and maybe you're saying:

> "But that's just the point, it could lead towards other insights within my life? What if I'm not sure I want insights about myself? What if that's too scary? You want me to be vulnerable! I don't know if I can do that!"

Fully understandable. For many people, it's not that they can't come up with topics to discuss. It's the whole idea of *how* to go about discussing those topics when you haven't been fully aware of them to this point in life. How do you discuss something that you're not sure how to put into words yourself?

Your goals must be worth it.

Trying to find the words as to what's in your subconscious or what's "holding you back" will be tough. Finding the words to *describe what your goals are* will be easier. Start there and focus there:

- What are the fitness goals you want?
- Why is it you want those goals?
- Keep working with your counselor if the words don't come to you easily.

How do I find a good counselor?

I personally have had some bartenders in my life that are good at making a certain drink just the way I like it. Plus, they do a great job of balancing professionalism, attentiveness and friendliness while maintaining the drink/food orders of other customers in a crowded facility.

I've had barbers who not just cut hair but are great at casual conversations (not too intrusive, not too superficial, just right) to pass the time on sports, dating, or current events.

Not every bartender or barber I've had has been great in all aspects. Some are great at making drinks or cutting hair and aren't good at the social aspect at all and vice versa. Some that are great for me, aren't great for everyone.

Overall, our culture is completely used to the industries of bartending and hair grooming. So, we'll continue to seek them out when we don't have a current "good one". We'll always keep looking until we find one that we like.

Currently, our culture may not do that with counseling. And all too often the result is: If we get one that isn't a great fit for us? Or we have a bad experience? Or even if we hear about a bad/lukewarm experience? Poof, we're gone, the whole industry can be discredited.

In terms of the counselor. It's not just about what he or she can give back to you. Many times, it's about what you can talk-through yourself out loud. Even when you're fumbling for the right words, the actual exercise of speaking issues or frustration or patterns out loud can be helpful on its own. It could be the mechanism you use to figure it out yourself. Especially when you focus on your goals.

But without a *trusted space* to be able to speak out loud it stays inside our heads. And inside our heads is the problem in the first place.

Stigmas

Finding a *trusted space*. I don't just mean the physical space where you have a conversation with a counselor. The emotional safe space is still a literal place to be able to open up while still figuring out the words to say. Especially in those first few sessions.

But there are pre-existing roadblocks for many of us. Stigmas such as:

> "That whole system is a joke. Doctors, nurses, hospitals, paperwork, insurance companies. It's all one big scam."

A large portion of our country doesn't trust going to their regular doctor. Not just because of avoiding hearing "bad news". But because of a long-standing mistrust of the overall system. Especially in areas of this country that haven't traditionally had quality healthcare readily available. When any system doesn't serve the needs of the people, the people feel as through the system just doesn't care about them.

"I don't want to talk to a stranger."

Our goals must be bigger than our fears. Speaking to a person who does not know you means they are not biased by any previous relationships or incidents with you. They can give you an unbiased opinion for advice or listening ear on your issues. People you already have an existing relationship with could be biased by just that – the nature of your relationship with them.

> "I only want to talk about what's going on wrong with me right now. Not divulge more information about other things that could be wrong overall".

The short-term goal of *"why can't I stop eating/doing XYZ when I know I want to lose weight"* is answered by looking at memories SAM sees or remembers that you may not. Remember, we need to hear from SAM to discuss what's wrong. Not just us.

> "I already talk to people about what's on my mind."

Going to a therapist/counselor and talking about "your problems" is viewed as degrading in many parts of this country (especially in lower-income areas, where it may be needed the most).

It's not just being vulnerable, because many of us will indeed open up to our favorite bartenders and barbers (it wasn't an accident we brought them up). And for many, that seems well enough. Our friends, family members, bartenders and barbers may have the best intentions, but are they aware of the detailed connections between our mind, our emotions, and our actions? Professional counselors are.

> "And doesn't going to a shrink make me look crazy? People will think I'm crazy! Heck, I will think: Maybe I am crazy!"

Mental illness versus emotional health. Mental disorders like Borderline Personality Disorder, Schizophrenia, OCD, Bi-polar and PTSD makes it seem like something is *"wrong with those people"*. And then we don't want to be lumped in with "them". The stigma of a psych ward with drooling patients or some person walking down the street talking loudly to themselves is a stereotype that comes to mind.

A *psychologist office*, where we sit down and talk and a *psychiatrist office* where we get help with psych meds, seems the same: Places where *crazy people* go! They're not the same, and even our judgment on "them" is unfounded.

> "Plus, that crap doesn't even work."

The whole concept of sitting down and talking *"about your problems"* to some other person who is not your bartender or barber is just too far-fetched for many humans. To compare it to a car mechanic, it's hard to believe in the concept that a counselor can "fix" you and put you back out on the road "better".

> "Those people won't understand me."

We all think our problems are unique. And to an extent they are. But we'd be surprised how our individual problems fall under the umbrella of common fears and insecurities. Meaning, the counselor/therapist can help us by relating through their experiences of helping others.

Even if the counselor hasn't walked in your shoes, he/she can still help us walk our path more confidently than we have before due to their *education and experience*.

Those *two factors* are also the biggest differences between a professional counselor and our comfort zone counselors of our friends, family, bartenders, and barbers.

One: Education.

Professionally counselors can tell the difference between SAM wanting ice cream because it's a deep reminder of past good times (which your comfort zone counselors might be able to figure out) or self-sabotaging your diet goals with ice cream is fueled by a deeper wound of SAM being told when you were young that you're not *worthy of accomplishments*. The 2nd revelation is why you *don't really want to lose weight* and it's not just about ice cream.

Two: Experience.

Counselors can also reassure you that you're not the only one that feels that way about good times or self-sabotage.

> "Wait I thought we all had our individual attachments to our individual issues? You said butter pecan ice cream attachment is different for you than me. What happened to that? Now you're saying we all have the same issues?"

The experiences counselors have in talking to other people gives them the credibility to let you know that while your experiences in your life are unique, there are broader sentiments that many other humans who have been in similar situations feel as well. Your specific situation is still unique, but others have been through similar situations and the counselor can reassure you that it's *not just you* that feels or responds in this fashion.

This can all take some time. That is, more than one sit down conversation. Which of itself is another "outside the comfort zone" activity. SAM doesn't like new habits. If going to a therapist, doctor, trainer, or gym is new: Then our subconscious is still protecting us from things we don't know – which is why forming new habits is difficult. Just like restaurant lighting and social media algorithms, knowing this information consciously can help.

You've been in the passenger seat for a long time, you may not switch over to full time driving for a while. Your "bad" eating habits (which again, aren't the problem themselves, it's your emotional attachment to those bad habits) have been in place for a while and you've been viewing "the sacrifice" of those bad things for an even longer time. With your new attitude of viewing things as fun, take your time and view this as a fun learning experience.

"Fun" in terms of learning to drive the car. Not just ride along in the passenger seat. The view out of the front windshield is the same. Let's enjoy it.

Examining our subconscious and then Discussing our self-awareness and self-regulation can help us with our own fitness journeys. But we can do more utilizing our knowledge.

We can Impact the systems around us. That's our next section. Let's start in Vegas!

SECTION 4

Impact Health Systems

CHAPTER 11

Information Overload

JUGGLING GYMS, DIETS AND SCHEDULES

February 2006. 8am.

Mandalay Bay hotel, Las Vegas Nevada.

Opening session of the week-long National Sales Meeting for my employer, a mid-sized, Massachusetts based pharmaceutical company.

The C-suite level management team, along with a hired professional speaker are at center stage. They are collectively hosting all company-employed sales and scientific personnel from every corner of the country. Their goal is to whip the 1,200 or so representatives into an excitement-level frenzy. This is the only time in the calendar year where we are all in one location, one room.

The lighting up on stage and throughout this enormous conference ballroom is pulsing along with the instrumental music. Adding to the sensory overload are huge floor-to-ceiling video screens in case your seat is too far from the stage to see details. Everyone is out of their seats and clapping along. At various points during this production, the folks on stage give our key competitors brief mentions, if only to solicit the formulaic passionate boos from the crowd.

Then they give shouts out to the teams from the "West Coast Region".

Huge applause.

"The East Coast Team!"

Ravenous cheering.

"Where's my South Team?"

Delirious clapping.

"Midwest. Are you in here?"

Feverish shouting.

If you didn't know any better, you'd think you would have arrived at the start of a rock concert for an internationally famous band on their initial tour night.

But it's 8am, round one, day one. We're just loosening up the cork on our week-long bottle of a meeting. We'll be here all week, in much more somber, focused breakout rooms around the hotel conference center. We'll be trained in how to sell to our healthcare customers, how to compare our specific products versus our specific competitors in *very* specific health-care commercial market disease-states and how to analyze our territories for maximum efficiency.

These meetings start daily at breakfast 6:30-7:45am. You had better be in your seat at 7:50am at the latest, because they will start on time at 8am sharp. (And trust me, despite there being 1,200 people, *you will be noticed* if you specifically are not in your seat promptly. Because your manager is keeping track of his/her 8-10 people.) Better to arrive at all sessions 10-15 minutes early.

The schedule is grueling: Breakout rooms from 9 to noon. Lunch. Afternoon sessions from 1 to 4:30-5pm. And it's not over then. They'll give us time to change clothes and visit our individual hotel rooms before being back in the lobby between 5:30 - 6pm for our evening event.

Evening events are scheduled until 9 or 10pm. They have themes, and occasionally the company rents out an actual concert venue (Grand Ole Opry in Nashville, Hard Rock café in Orlando) or just envelopes a whole wing of a resort/hotel (Swan and Dolphin Disney or Gaylord in Dallas). Evening affairs are "fun" to help you bond with your teammates. You will absolutely need your teammates as a resource when you're back out there on your own in the vast geographical solitude of your territory.

Back to the 2006 Mandalay Bay. It's now 9pm. We're at their closing evening events. Amid the exquisite buffet tables and open bars scattered throughout this gigantic banquet all is an indescribable ice-sculpture-and-trapeze-artist backdrop. The meetings are usually information overload, and this room is sensory overload.

In general, company meetings like this one are copy and paste throughout the pharmaceutical and lab-diagnostic industries. These firms emotionally charge their employees in larger assembly meetings, then functionally pump their personnel with information during those somber, smaller breakout groups. You will be expected to absorb and utilize scientific training, software resources and territory data.

Again, it's all information overload. And unless you head out on your own at 9, 10 pm or arrive to the host city a day or two early, you *rarely* get any personal time to sightsee in Vegas, Nashville, Dallas, LA, Orlando, etc. where the meeting is held. Sound like a lot? These companies can't afford to *not* throw everything at you. Why?

One. They need you to be fired up. Not just to take on this grueling workweek but to still have passion for the job long after you're back home and alone in your territory.

Two. You're going to be up against: Large hospital conglomerates with their highly business-oriented workforce *and* individual billing specialists who sift their way through an alphabet-soup of government and commercial insurance entities.

Three. You are facing the apathy of physicians and nurse practitioners who have their own daily/weekly numbers to achieve. These healthcare employees are frequently squeezed for time by the metrics set forth by their parent company, leaving them with a picogram of patience for your products or personality. Not to mention, these offices get visits from representatives from all types of companies, most of which are not your direct market competitors, but still take up the office's collective time.

As a company, your employer has real money invested in you while real stock investors have placed money into it. All entities involved are expecting a financial return on their investments. Therefore, the company needs you to be emotionally attached to your local goals, your manager's regional goals and the company metrics as well. That's why they are pouring all they can into you here in Vegas today.

This is the opposite of that conference in Philadelphia.

Meaning: the emotion of apathy, which was exhibited by the patient's families at that conference cannot be allowed to germinate within you. These companies not only need to deposit this vast amount of information into you, but they also can't *afford* for you to be indifferent in the slightest.

This meeting in Vegas is also the *opposite* of what you face during your individual fitness journey.

The parallel: In your fitness journey, there is also information overload. And while personal trainers and dieticians and health care

professionals and online gurus all swear that they are here to help –
that's just the point! Where do you even get started finding the right
people to help you in the beginning?

No one is guiding you through your journey by placing you in a room
full of 1,200 pulsating people then breakout rooms of 10-50 people
to show you, step by step, how you'll get this done all to hold you
accountable once you get back to the solitude of your day-to-day life.
No one.

Re-emphasize that last part about accountability. Just like you had
better be on time (*early is better!*) to every one of these meetings this
week in Vegas, you had better bring in those sales numbers during
this upcoming 2006 calendar year or they will find someone who
can. Again, these companies literally can't afford for you to fail them.

The contrast: No entity is currently holding you accountable for
your fitness goals with the threat of financial distress to them if
you don't reach your goals. Even our stripper from Chapter 7, with
supplementary earnings hanging in the balance, could not vanquish
her subconscious' desires.

We're done here in Vegas. Fly home safely.

The REDI Network creates a discussion
platform for delicate topics.

This chapter shows how to
Impact the overwhelming
information we face on our
Journeys towards fitness.

Unlike the 8am opening session in Vegas, so many people on their fitness journey aren't exactly certain where to begin.

The questions start internally. You might have had a similar conversation with yourself about all the things you'll need to start this journey. The conversation frequently goes:

> "I guess I'll join a gym. I'll ask my friends about what type of diets worked for them then I'll look up one or two of those and I'll be all set.
>
> Wait, what foods do I eat before I go workout? And how close to working out should I eat? And what am I supposed to do in the gym? Lifting looks too intimidating, and I don't want to bulk up like that.
>
> I'll just do the treadmill. No, I'll take their cycle class. No, I'll do the treadmill after all because I don't want to be in a group class with people looking at me while I struggle.
>
> Wait, when I go to the grocery store, am I supposed to eat all this spinach before it goes bad in 4 days? Maybe I'll get a meal-prep company to make meals.
>
> Do I need some protein powder?
> Or just the shakes?
> Does any of it taste good?
> Is potato salad a vegetable?
> Are you kidding me, these diets want me to give up bread?
> I love bread! I already see I'm going to hate all this!"

It's no wonder so many fitness dreams cause more stress than results. It's a lot of information to juggle. Think about each one of these

3 information items and how taxing it can be to sort all of it out individually as opposed to a company doing literal pyrotechnics in Vegas to keep its employees emotionally engaged.

Information item 1: Workout facilities

You must sort through the huge range of gyms, yoga studios, stationary bike facilities, cross-training services, step classes etc. How many of these do we have in our country?

"With 36,180 health clubs as of 2015, the United States has more fitness centers than any other country in the world. Brazil has a similarly high number as it is home to over 30,000 fitness centers. All other countries in the world have fewer than 9,000 fitness clubs." (Gough, 2017)

So, we have the most facilities on the planet. Excellent. How active are we with those memberships? Are we turning those into better health?

We acquire gym memberships, and they aren't fully being utilized. Those aren't just wasted opportunities to get in shape, it's wasted money. Also, according to Finder.com research, 5.1 million Americans waste a total of $1.8 billion down the drain on unused gym memberships every single year.

"Over half of all Americans (53%) pay for a gym membership, even if they aren't using it. Of those with an active membership, roughly 41 million (49.9%) actually get to the gym at least twice a week. A further 24.2% make it to the gym at least once a week. More people have never used their membership (6.3%) than those who either use their membership once a month (5.8%) or less than once a month (5.4%)." (McDermott, 2019)

The good news. We can **R**ealize the source of our frustrations by **E**xamining our subconscious to **D**iscuss why as individuals can figure out which gym, which membership would be best for us. We Impact these systems of facilities with our own emotional intelligence. Not only does this keep us from feeling frustrated like "Tom" in chapter 8, but we also won't feel the arrogance on the other side of that same coin once we reach our fitness goals.

Information item 2: Our Diet Plans

The Keto diet, Mediterranean diet, Plant Based diet, South Beach Diet, Flexitarian Diet.

Meal plans fit in here as well. Because who wants to constantly grocery shop? BistroMD, Medifast, Weight watchers, Plate-Joy, Beach Body and Trifecta!

"An estimated 45 million Americans go on a diet each year. Americans spend $33 billion each year on weight loss dietary products." (Harfman, 2021)

Seems like this entire industry is filling in the gaps so that we don't have to do an extensive internet search. All manners of services will just deliver food to the house or tell us what to eat each day, each meal.

Total: with Supplements, Gym member ships, Gym clothes, Meal plans, Nutritional advice (meal plans) and personal trainers. It all adds up to $155 /per month per American per Arabella Olgivie at us.myprotein.com.

The good news. Our emotional journey towards self-awareness will leave us able to manage our time and our outlook towards diet. I still wish to apologize to my Chapter 7 stripper client for not knowing this at the time of her tenacious workouts.

Information item 3: Internet & Experts

The internet has endless amounts of Tik Tok and YouTube workout videos. Dietary Gurus with glittering websites. Instagram fitness celebrities. Jillian Michaels. Shaun Thompson. Billy Blanks. Even Jane Fonda and Richard Simmons videos are still accessible.

We have access to so much information it's almost sensory overload. Where to we even start to sort out all this information?

All these experts have different ideas on what to eat, when to eat it, establishing goals, writing down workout routines, and tracking results.

Only, if your subconscious is not on board with this seemingly insurmountable accumulation of information it will either be rare that results happen, or it will be a struggle every day to stay on course.

The total combination of negotiating workout facilities, adjusting our eating habits, and digesting the vast sums of information isn't to be taken lightly.

Having set plans is still incredibly important.

- Part of the fitness journey is your personal research. It will be time invested in yourself. Know the gym, diet and/or guru that's best for you. We can't just start The Keto/Atkins Diet or any other without knowing the pros and cons.
- It isn't just going to a workout facility that will lead to changes. What are your goals when there? Are you going to the gym to lift for bulk? To increase your cardiovascular capacity? To strengthen and stabilize a muscle-group that has been weak-spot? Being specific is critical.

- Understanding nutrition is again all about why a certain diet plan is right for you as an individual. How will it help you not just to reach your goals, but to increase your knowledge of how your body responds to certain foods or food groups or portion sizes. Coordinating those foods with your exercise routine at your specific stage of your journey is paramount. If you're losing 100+ pounds, then most of your weight loss will come from your adjusted diet. If you're losing 10 pounds, then it's a balance of training and diet. Know all of it with as much detail as possible. Absolutely.
- The information glut needs to be refined for your unique goals. Your specific path.

All this planning and comprehension of the physical attributes and activities can't be minimized whatsoever.

However, without *full* knowledge of the specific emotional obstacles have been in your way: None of these matters for the long haul.

Digesting all this information helps us Impact the fitness systems that are all around us in this country. There is another system that Impacts our fitness dilemma: The institutions of research. And what better place to visit next than the National Institutes of Health.

Pack your bags, we're Leaving Las Vegas like it's 1995. We're headed back east to discuss how obesity stresses the body versus how societal pressures stress obese bodies.

CHAPTER 12

Obesity versus Health
THE BIOMARKERS OF FAT-SHAMING

May 2018. National Institutes of Health, Bethesda, Maryland.

In stark contrast to the opening session in Las Vegas, the unpretentious vendor fair on the NIH campus is taking place inside a large provisional tent sprawled across a vacated, unevenly surfaced parking lot near building 10. There are no pulsating light shows, no ice-sculptures, no hired speakers. There are indeed several dozen vendors presenting a spectrum of technologies and services to hundreds of science lab workers amidst this makeshift venue.

First, you and I will find our designated area under the tent. Then we'll drape our pre-made company logo tablecloth over a provided folding table. We'll place our demonstration machines and samples on the tabletop and meticulously arrange our paraphernalia and information for other products not on display but still part of our research lab distribution portfolio.

Now we'll stand behind our table.

And wait.

Customers peruse the entire area under the tent in their free time. Occasionally you and I will have a dozen people at our table. More than occasionally, we'll have crickets. When folks meander towards our table and express a direct interest/need for our equipment/reagents? We close the deal! We make agreements to ship our products or the products of our abundant partnered distributors to them ASAP! Don't look now, but our competitors are only a few aisles away and they're zealous to peddle as well. All vendors standing behind our tables under this tent have quarterly and yearly metrics and quotas for which we're held accountable. None of us are here for charity work.

During these interactions with lab personnel, you and I, as Life Science Specialists, are working on more than just transactions for today. We need to become acquainted with the obstacles and objectives of their protocols. The necessities of today may not be all they need in their next scientific objectives. Also, if we build genuine rapport through our personas and expertise, they will not merely become customers, but refer us to their peers – not our company – us. You and me.

Like people, Like People.

But alas, what we're doing here today is not merely enough. Yes, we're building bonds with scientists at shows. Yes, on other days of the week, we're visiting labs here at NIH and at local research universities and biotech and pharmaceutical research facilities across a multi-state region. And I wish I could tell you that the resulting sales of electroporators, ELISA kits, PCR sequencers, flow cytometers, and western blot detection reagents moved the needle in terms of our advancements along the fitness battle versus obesity in America.

We help... but...

Here, across this NIH campus, we constantly melt minds with experts who work at the National Institutes of Diabetes & Digestive Kidney & Kidney Diseases - NIDDK. They absolutely need our products and proficiency, but our combined effect on the obesity conundrum is well... limited.

Same for the exceptional researchers from Heart Lung and Blood Institutes - NHLBI. We have items that can assist their work. But there's only so much we can do.

These two divisions weren't random inclusions. They're both part of the NIH Obesity Research Task Force: Established to understand the inherent genetic, biological, environmental, and behavioral factors that contribute to obesity.

Several hours have passed. Our time is up under this tent for today. This vendor fair is over. I truly thank you for your work at our table. As we break down the equipment, fold away the tablecloth and pack up the paraphernalia, I want you to know our efforts on behalf of our company and our collaborative discussions with these researchers were not completely in vain.

Alas, for you and me, as we matriculate towards our cars, our discussions today were restricted to the physics, chemistry, and biology of the subject matter. However, the Obesity in America battle isn't just waged in gyms, yoga studios, internet fad diets nor limited to these scientific labs at NIH.

You know who didn't come to our table? The folks from the NIH center for Biotechnology Information. Their psychology-based research documenting the *stress* of being judged (fat shaming) by *society and self* is just as paramount in this battle as the cellular and molecular causations being studied by our direct clients on this campus. We had nothing from our vast list of products to help with their studies on these emotional implications.

Good teamwork today. Drive home safely.

The REDI Network creates a discussion platform for delicate topics.

Chapter 12 shows how we can Impact the systems of the medical community by addressing fat shaming, fatness alone and biomarkers.

Allow me to transition back to that April 2023 cruise out of Miami. I put in a **pause** for people triggered by certain terms: Fat Shaming and Body Positivity. Let's walk right back to that buffet and allow me to elaborate further.

Do you know what I *really* saw on this vessel? Fat people feverishly gobbling up a greasy, gluttonous buffet on a Floating Golden Corral. Do you know what I really felt? Disgust. Disappointment. Disdain.

Stay with me and hold that sentiment while thinking back to that pharmaceutical drug closet from Chapter 6 and let me continue to reflect. Two things can be true at the same time about Dr. Smith. She absolutely was lamenting how her patient didn't receive/take-seriously what she was advising about losing weight. You know what else I heard in her voice now that I think about it through the lens of the Body Positivity movement or the principles of Fat Shaming? It wasn't just frustration I overheard; it was disdain and disappointment.

Now bring that held sentiment from the cruise buffet and the tone of Dr. Smith together and let's add one more industry to the list of industries that are potentially emotionally sabotaging our fitness endeavors by manipulating our subconscious: The medical community itself. Because that sentiment of disdain isn't limited to "Dr. A Smith, general practitioner".

The medical community mirrors us. All of us. For all those obese people that I've seen in my decades working in doctor's offices, I still was blown away by that multi-decked, oceanic human ecosystem of food consumption called a cruise. And remember, it wasn't just me with this reaction after witnessing that spectacle. The owner of the yoga studio shared the same reactions after her cruise experience years prior. In the exact moments when she shared her story - days before my departure - I couldn't relate to the smorgasbord spectacle she was describing. To be clear, I was *looking forward* to the food. I was confused by her comments. Then I saw it. And it wasn't the food. It was the people eating the food.

Humans judge and shame other humans for being overweight. The effect of that judgment is now being quantified - and not just by NIH researchers in Biotechnology Information.

"There's also a growing body of research that indicates that health risks we typically associate with being fat may be driven by fat people's experiences of bias and discrimination." (Williams, 2020)

"Many common anti-obesity efforts are unintentionally complicit in contributing to weight stigma. Standard medical advice for weight loss focuses on taking individual responsibility and exerting willpower ('eat less, exercise more'). In this context, a little shame is seen as motivation to change diet and activity behaviors. Nevertheless, this approach perpetuates stigmatization, as higher-weight individuals already engage in self-blame and feel ashamed of their weight." (Tomiyama, 2018)

Like People Like People. The opposite can be true as well. And this Impact shows up in lab diagnostics.

The Biology of Obesity
Example 1: Type 2 diabetes.

Earlier today at the vendor fair, our friends from the Institutes of Diabetes and Digestive and Kidney diseases came by our table. Their research on the relationship between obesity and how your body can no longer regulate its blood glucose levels is well documented.

Let's examine the current statistics linking obesity to this disease state.

"The lifetime diabetes risk in men older than 18 years increases from 7% to 70% when BMI increases from less than 18.5 kg/m to more than 35 kg/m. Similarly, the lifetime diabetes risk in females increases from 12% to 74% with the same BMI values." (Yashi, 2023)

Add to that are facts from the American Diabetes Association:

- 80% of people who have diabetes are overweight.
- One in 3 in this country will have diabetes by 2050. Not only is this disease-state increasing, but it is also projected to continue rising.
- The American Diabetes Association sees more money being spent on this disease because more people are being diagnosed with it.

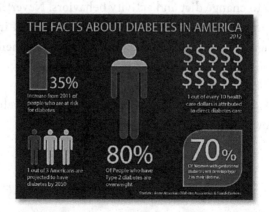

The takeaways aren't just linking obesity to the health risk of diabetes, the statistics show this epidemic is *increasingly* affecting our population and corresponding health care costs.

The Biology of Obesity
Example 2: C-Reactive Protein

The commonly screened biomarker: C-Reactive Protein is used to detect inflammation. CRP levels assist in diagnosing cardiovascular issues (heart disease, high blood pressure) and auto-immune disorders (lupus, rheumatoid arthritis).

"Long-term CRP elevation can lead to adult-onset obesity. CRP can also provoke a broad adjustment in the innate immune system and energy expenditure system. CRP may be a new therapeutic target for obesity and its complications." (Li, 2020)

The Biology of Obesity
Example 3: Trends over time.

Staying with the shifting cardiological effects of obesity in America; a study published in the American Heart Association in 2007 studied the trends in High Blood Pressure (HBP) within children and adolescents. The researchers knew that many of the issues we see with adults begin in childhood.

They took a representative sample of 8 to 17-year-old subjects over the previous 40 years and the impact of obesity increased on the trends in the past 10 years.

Explicitly, the trends were:

- Elevated blood pressure has been on the rise since the late 1980s, after a long period of decreasing trend.

- The increase in obesity accounts for the upward trend of HBP.
- Racial/ethnic trends in BP followed racial/ethnics trends in obesity.

The 1980s. Many of the discussion points in the previous chapters regarding the food, restaurant and television industries transformed drastically in breadth and scope during that time frame. Our obesity rates, and health implications skyrocketed then as well.

So did our judgement.

How Societal Disdain for Obesity:
Manifests in Biomarkers

Long before the 1980s, our society had disdain for "Fat People".

"In a classic study performed in the late 1950s, 10- and 11-year-olds were shown six images of children and asked to rank them in the order of which child they 'liked best'.

The six images included:

- A 'normal' weight child,
- An 'obese' child,
- A child in a wheelchair,
- One with crutches and a leg brace,
- One with a missing hand,
- Another with a facial disfigurement.

Across six samples of varying social, economic, and racial/ethnic backgrounds from across the United States, the child with obesity was ranked last." (Richardson, 1961)

We've been viewing "Fat People" as unpleasing to our eyes for generations. Our society has sought, celebrated, and marketed our toned & fit male physiques and female figures. Antithetically, we've scorned, criticized, and maligned chubby, flabby humans. Why?

Because, unlike the *other* children available for our visual review in that 1961 report, we surmise that being overweight is indeed under your control. Therefore, if you're obese, it's *your* fault that you're this way. From there we judge you as lazy, lacking willpower and worthy of our disdain. It makes "us" better than "you". And you sense that. Which brings us back to the science of stress on the same disease states studied by our customers from the vendor fair.

"The mere perception of oneself as being overweight, across the BMI spectrum (i.e., even among individuals at a 'normal' BMI), is prospectively associated with biological markers of poorer health, including unhealthy blood pressure, C-reactive protein, HDL cholesterol, triglycerides, glucose, and HbA1c levels. Collectively, these findings suggest that stigma attached to being 'overweight' is a significant yet unrecognized agent in the causal pathway from weight status to health." (Tomiyama, 2018)

Now that we've listed all this data, the next time we attend a vendor fair, we'll have to encourage our current customers to collaborate with the growing psychological studies affecting the biochemistry of obesity. Because the biomarker levels we specifically attribute to poor health outcomes are directly prompted by our social stigmas; not just our diets, gym-habits, or sedentary lifestyle.

Therefore, it is even more critical that we find the underlying subconscious emotional dilemmas that each single individual is facing while aggressively rejecting the stigmatization of any patient or person for their outward appearance. If this is truly about fitness, and not fat, then our country's health depends on this delineation.

This topic re-emphasizes focus of the REDI Network:

- **R**ealize the source of individual outlooks and biases.
- **E**xplore our subconscious to become more self-aware. Explore our individual attachments to corporate entities' emotional manipulation.
- **D**iscuss self-awareness with others, without apprehension of being wrong or right about previous conceptions.
- **I**mpact the systems around us. In this book, these systems are the fitness and healthcare communities.

An additional example of that **I**mpact: The yoga studio where I instruct H.I.I.T. Hot Pilates prides itself on being highly accepting of all people, no matter what their background is or where they are along their current fitness journeys. Every single day, the studio's community of instructors, staff and members absolutely exude the desired palpable vibration of acceptance. However, is the all-are-welcome culture limited to the physical space within the walls of the facility?

We may subconsciously alleviate judgment of overweight or obese individuals when they are physically present at our studio. Again, humans for generations have viewed "fat people" as exhibiting a lack of control over their lives. Well, when you're at the studio, you're "doing something about it". You're taking control. And that makes you *so* welcome inside that studio from the moment you walk in.

But if you are the exact same overweight person and you're holding your plate with one hand while piling on more food with the other hand at the all-you-can-eat buffet on a cruise ship... then the exact same humans who populate that hot yoga studio may have the subconscious reaction of judgment. It's not anything we're consciously aware of in the moment it's happening.

Our medical community is not exempt from this paradox. The publications cited in this chapter *illuminate* not only the stress felt by obese individuals in the presence of a professional community designed to aid their health, but the *resulting* biochemical implications of that judgement.

Make no mistake. There are still serious health consequences with "fatness" and fatness alone. Our line in the sand should be drawn between the biological repercussions and the psychological ramifications of the biomarkers detailed in these previous pages. Meaning, individuals whose biomarkers are still exceeding standards for poor health outcomes, should still own a personal responsibility to physically alter their lifestyles.

Go back to my dear friend from Chapter 9. She has stated - for the purposes of being quoted in this book - that while she indeed judges *herself*, she has not felt judged by anyone in her healthcare facilities on her visits.

Solution for her: Emotional Intelligence can help her self-awareness and her outlook on her fitness journey. If she is verifiably biometrically healthy, developing a strong sense of self-love by disregarding society's generational fixations on what her body *should* look like can alleviate self-judgment. She may not need to lose as much weight as her original goal from that chapter's story in order to be *healthy*.

Alas, my dear friend is also a prime example of our country-wide biometric reality:

- She is pre-diabetic.
- She takes medication for her idiopathic intracranial hypertension which her physician has stated could be negated by losing weight.
- She also needs to lose weight for a non-emergency hernia.

Despite these biological issues, which should be motivation, she has battled weight loss for two decades now.

As we shall examine further in the next chapter, our current national obesity trends are all pointing in the wrong direction. And that will affect more than just our patient-by-patient biomarker levels at the doctor's office. It affects all of us. Yes, even citizens who are not overweight. Yes, even citizens who are not obese or remotely out of shape.

For the record. I still had a good time on that cruise. It was fun! Because: Do you know what else they had in vast locations spread throughout the ship that was right up *my* alley?

Bars.

I absolutely had the alcohol-wristband package. All you can drink. I uh, sure hope no one from uh, the hot yoga studio or the uh, NIH vendor fair was there judging me (looks both ways, takes another sip).

CHAPTER 13

Mississippi Money

FUTURE ECONOMICS OF OBESITY

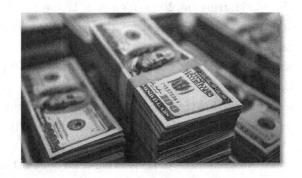

January 2035.

570 East Woodrow Wilson Drive, Jackson Mississippi.

Chief medical officer Dr. Justin Turner and Chief of Community Health Victor Sutton, Ph.D. are meeting with the soon-to-be-retired Dr. Daniel Edney from his position as the State of Mississippi Health Officer. These three are joined by others from the MSDH Administration. Their concerns are not limited to the ranking of the state from a health perspective, and hence, they joined in this meeting by participants not hailing from The Magnolia State.

This year, Mississippi Medicaid and Medicare have reached their financial breaking points for funding while trying to stay ahead of the obesity crisis. Since 2023, the year after Dr. Edney started in his position, the great state of Mississippi had strengthened its position as the direst health care state.

Since 2023:

- Mississippi has gone from 13.3% (the highest in the country) (Harrington, 2023) of its over-20 population with diabetes to 19%.
- The adult obesity rate has risen from 41.2% (The highest in the country) (Harrington, 2023) to 48.9%.
- The percentage of adults over the age of 20 with diabetes was 13.3.%. (Harrington, 2023) It's now at 18.6%.
- Adults who don't exercise regularly 36.9% (the highest in the nation) (Harrington, 2023)is now 39%.
- Percentage of adults with limited access to healthy foods: 11.4% (2nd highest) (Harrington, 2023) to 15%.
- Median household income: $49,111 (the lowest in the nation) (Harrington, 2023) Has only increased to $53,000.

This last point - household income - is as big of an issue as the health metrics above it. And for that reason, also present in this meeting are members of the advisory board of the Peter G. Peterson foundation.

They have flown down from New York City with their Healthcare Reform team. This foundation stated, "in 2021, the U.S. devoted 18 percent of its economy to healthcare". (Peterson, n.d.) Now, in 2035, this figure has jumped to 23% - almost one-quarter of our American economy to our health.

Why is an economics-driven, NYC think-tank meeting with the Mississippi Department of Health? For the current situation in 2035, the medical experts and economic pundits need to conjure a model to fix this state's woes. For us back in 2024, we all can benefit as a nation using their plan.

The consequence of the meeting requires the somber immediacy of any patient these doctors-turned-administrators have treated. Fixing the Mississippi economic entanglement from the obesity crises is essential. The rest of us benefiting would be remarkable. However, as we sit here in 2035, it's the world economy which is truly in need of overhaul from its struggles with obesity.

The REDI Network creates a discussion platform for delicate topics.

This chapter details the Impact of the severe trends in obesity and the long-term economic effects.

2035. The global obesity dilemma has consumed the world's population. Here are the sobering projections:

World Obesity Economics

"51% of the world's population — or roughly 4 billion people — are expected to be overweight (BMI over 25) or obese (BMI over 30) by 2035, a significant jump from the 38% of the population who were overweight or obese in 2020. the economic impact of a high BMI could reach $4.32 trillion annually". (WorldObesity.org, 2023)

"Roughly 3 percent of global GDP — about as much as the economy grows in a year or the same impact as the Covid-19 pandemic in 2020". (WorldObesity.org, 2023)

It's not just the money spent.

It's not merely the percentage of the budgets.

It's the worldwide trends. The direction of every graph, every chart, every tangible metric show we're headed into an obesity-driven economic catastrophe with no current ideas on how to reverse these trends.

"Worldwide: Not a single country has seen a decline in obesity prevalence since 1975." (Belluz, 2023)

National Obesity Economics

The United States: Ranked higher than any other major country on earth for obesity. We spend tons of money and effort on gyms and diets. How does our culture and lack of individual emotional intelligence and fitness show up in our economic statistics:

How much do we spend?

"The United States spends nearly three times as much on healthcare as other advanced nations, but unfortunately our system rarely provides better health outcomes." (Peterson, n.d.)

"Looking ahead, researchers have estimated that by 2030, if obesity trends continue unchecked, obesity-related medical costs alone could rise by $48 to $66 billion a year in the U.S.". (Chan, 2024)

"We estimate the total costs in 2018 to be $1.39 trillion, consisting of $370 billion in direct costs for medical treatment for each condition and indirect costs of $1.02 trillion for lost workdays, calculated as lost employee output. The total estimated cost of obesity equals 6.76 percent of GDP in 2018 compared to 5.57 percent in 2014". (Lopez, 2020)

What are the trends?

"The share of total health care spending of non-institutionalized adults that is devoted to treating obesity-related illness has risen from 20.6 percent in 2005 to 27.5 percent in 2010 to 28.2 percent in 2013". (Beiner, 2017)

"The total direct medical costs of obesity in adults more than doubled during the study period, from $124.2 in 2001 to $260.6 billion in 2016. In 2016, $139.4 billion was paid by private health insurance, $57.9 billion was paid by public health insurance programs, and $20.0 billion was paid out of pocket by patients for obesity-related care." (Cawley, 2021)

"One widely quoted estimate from Finkelstein and colleagues, based on data from the U.S. Medical Expenditure Panel Survey (MEPS), found that obesity was responsible for about 6 percent of medical costs in 1998, or about $42 billion (in 2008 dollars). By 2006, obesity was responsible for closer to 10 percent of medical costs—nearly $86 billion a year. Spending on obesity-related conditions accounted for an estimated 8.5 percent of Medicare spending, 11.8 percent of Medicaid spending, and 12.9 percent of private-payer spending." (Chan, 2024)

According to the CDC, obesity-related medical care costs the United States public $147 billion a year. Roughly half of all medical costs associated with obesity are financed by Medicare and Medicaid. In terms of government spending, the cost of treating obesity in our healthcare system is greater than what all US governments (federal, state, and local) combined to spend in a typical year. (USAFacts.org, 2020)

I'm not sure if the greater point from that last article is that:

- We spent $147 Billion on our obesity issues,

- The title itself. We dramatically increased our obesity rates in 50 short years. This goes back to the evolution of subliminal marketing for the industries we've discussed. Emotional manipulation of our subconscious began in the 1970s and 80s. Here are our results.
- Those rates went from 14% to almost 40%. That is an astronomical jump during *any* time frame!

Next. Our trends aren't just bad for current adults. Our children will continue to increase these trends.

A 2009 study published in the Journal of Health Affairs arising from the realization that obesity in adults can start as obesity in children can lead to increased hospitalizations and costs. That study (Leonardo Trasande, Yinghua Liu, George Fryar, Michael Weitzman) found a near-doubling of diagnosis of obesity by hospitals in the United States.

State Obesity Economics

All the above statistics reflect our national trends. Large differences exist across states, Cawley said. In 2015, states such as Arizona, California, Florida, New York, and Pennsylvania devoted five to six percent of their total medical expenditures to treating obesity-related illness, whereas North Carolina, Ohio and Wisconsin spent more than twice that — over 12 percent of all health care dollars in those states were used to treat obesity-related illness. (CornellUniversity, 2018)

From 2001-15, Kentucky and Wisconsin devoted over 20 percent of their Medicaid spending to obesity-related illness. In contrast, in New York, 10.9 percent of Medicaid spending was devoted to obesity-related illness. (CornellUniversity, 2018)

That Cornell University article shed some light on: Who exactly is more at risk for obesity-related health issues? There are other state by state and even county by county evidence to show obesity is growing more rapidly in under-educated, rural areas of our country.

"Overall, severe obesity cost state Medicaid programs almost $8 billion a year, ranging from $5 million in Wyoming to $1.3 billion in California." (Wang, 2015)

But does it matter which states are allocating more resources to combat our fitness crises than others? It does. We need to know where to focus our attention and resources for educating specific counties or municipalities. We can start with our friends at the beginning of this chapter in Mississippi.

Individual Obesity Economics

So, from world statistics, national metrics and state funding, all the numbers are showing increased spending and spiraling trends. But what affects us all directly is even more alarming: Health insurance premiums. Money out of all income.

Health insurance companies are charging your employer more per year to cover all these costs you just read. Our employers are feeling the crunch and passing along the responsibility to us. All of us.

Whether you are biomarker-fit or BMI obese. Hot Yoga studio member or Carnival Cruise buffet connoisseur. Largo Maryland stripper to Mississippi state chief medical officer. You are directly paying for our nation's fitness crises.

Yes, insurance companies are indeed measuring the body mass index (BMI) of every individual they cover and subsequently classifying anyone who meets their criteria as obese. However, they can't charge anyone more money in premiums.

Healthcare providers are using that classification using BMI to assess eligibility for various services. A BMI of 30 or above is classified as obese. Those services then can be made available for dietary counseling, weight-loss medications, and bariatric surgery.

While I'm not a fan of BMI as an indicator of health (I'd much prefer using Body Fat %) we simply need a metric that is used universally. Besides, no matter which metric we use, this data is pointing in the wrong direction.

But let's get back to your paycheck, your paystub, your direct deposit, your money.

Since the affordable care act dictates that insurance companies can't charge higher premiums for obesity, then the costs of our obesity crises come out of your check.

Employers take more from everyone's paycheck to cover these increasing costs (even indirect costs, because obese individuals take more time off, leading to less efficiency in the company's workforce) and that will continue to increase.

Numerous sources detail one of my favorite stat trends for this whole book: Not just for one state, not just for this country, but no *country* on the planet has seen a decrease in their obesity rates since 1975. Again, another indication of the time-phase when these metrics began to spike in the direction of fitness-related disaster.

"In 1988, health care premiums represented about 8% of a worker's total compensation, results showed. But by 2019, that number had jumped to nearly 18% of total compensation. If the cost of employer-sponsored insurance had remained at the same proportion as 1988, the average family could have earned $8,774 more in annual wages in 2019". (Thompson, 2024)

The more obese we get as a nation, the more comes out of our collective pay.

"Over 30 units of BMI, each one-unit BMI increase was associated with an additional cost of $253 (95% CI $167-$347) per person. Among adults, obesity was associated with $1,861 (95% CI $1,656-$2,053) excess annual medical costs per person, accounting for $172.74 billion (95% CI $153.70-$190.61) of annual expenditures." (Ward, 2021)

It doesn't matter if you or your neighbor is obese. Or if everyone on your block is obese or everyone on your block is in "elite" physical condition. The statistics show our state governments can't continue paying for our increasing rate of obesity-related illnesses and we can't continue to have more income going to pay for obesity-related health insurance premiums.

If the percentage of our overall population continues to grow at current trends, and the amount of money our government spends continues at a commensurate rate, it's not if but when will we be bankrupt on state levels due to this health crisis? By all estimations, that "when" is within the next 10-12 years.

Will we have to decide whether to fund public schools or pave roads & repair fallen bridges *or* pay for our obese population's hospital visits? This isn't just money coming out of your check. This is your tax money being spent and how it's allocated.

Politicians and citizens on a local, state, and federal level all debate constantly about whether to raise or lower our taxes. How much money can we save right now by just being healthier? To at least slow down the trends?

Which brings us back to that meeting in Jackson Mississippi with Drs. Turner, Sutton, and Edney. While the health metrics are dire, the lost wages from health care premiums extracting take home pay from millions of state residents - including the people in that room - is just as calamitous.

Mississippi residents already had the lowest median household income in the nation. Here in 2035, those residence are now having 24.8% of their pay taken out to cover health insurance premiums. The state that can least afford to have bad health outcomes is also the state that can least afford to have its citizens receiving less money.

Thanks again to the folks in Mississippi for meeting at a future time in a current place to solve our coming crises. They will be willing to do "whatever it takes" to change our culture and the direction of obesity's effect on their economy. Still, it's them being reactive to their circumstances, not proactive to the 2024 trends. That example lies in the future, we need to get ahead of the trends now.

I saw a whatever-it-takes mentality once and it was incredible, the impression was indelible. We need an example of how to always think proactively. Let's stay down in the deep south and drive a couple of states east from Mississippi and slide over to Georgia.

CHAPTER 14

Reactive vs Proactive

FIVE METHODS TOWARDS EQ

Fall 2003. Athens, Georgia.

The virtual drug screening program DOCK 4.0 had been designed to help optimize the serial process of drug screening. The goal of the software was to narrow down the vast amounts of available compounds without using robotics and reagents. My specific dissertation goal was to incorporate DOCK 4.0 as a method to help find new compounds that could disrupt the formation of a key protein in HIV.

My advisor took one single weekend to gulp down a 300+ page textbook on the UNIX/Linux applications of this software DOCK 4.0. I was just as *awed* by the intellectual prowess of my advisor on devouring complex information quickly as I was by the workout tenacity of that stripper from chapter 7.

Differentially, I considered myself and the rest of my lab-mates to be "smart people". But as a trained structural biologist and biochemistry professor, he supplemented his advanced aptitude with galvanization. He knew precisely what the information in that textbook – or any text of scientific or software material - would do for his career. His career is predicated on applying *his* knowledge to his lab full of graduate students and our various long-term experiments.

He could see the finished results of not only DOCK 4.0 to virtual drug screening of the HIV capsid protein, but also, he had the forthcoming wet-lab-bench work laid out in his mind and the ensuing submission to the appropriate scientific journal.

Just like the company meeting in Las Vegas – when they can't afford to not have you fired up after leaving their meeting, my advisor can't afford to not be **visionary**. He too has an investment.

He has a limited amount of time that his students in his lab can be under his direction for scientific projects. Therefore, if there is any information now and, in the future, (his conscious knows about the future) that he can apply to current or upcoming projects – he must retain that information in his long-term memory. Plus, like many humans in this field, he's a science geek (it's a loving term) and science geeks need to always know as much or more than other science geeks.

He is a fulcrum for the research interests within his lab in the same way research is the fulcrum for any academic community.

He **I**mpacts the systems of his department and university by consuming information just as *enthusiastically* as the crowds in the opening session in Vegas or my fellow cruise line vacationers. He doesn't need to **R**ealize the source or **E**xplore his subconscious and **D**iscuss his subconscious ruminations with professionals or peers.

He is also not being reactive. He is proactively Impacting the systems around him by seeking and storing knowledge. He isn't waiting for a problem to become too big to handle.

Contrastingly, our American culture does not function in this manner. I don't merely mean that we are capable of being a corporately manipulative, fat-shaming, decadent-reward-system culture that by and large, views emotional intelligence with a tepid response.

> The REDI Network creates a discussion platform for delicate topics.
>
> This chapter shows how we can Impact our apathetic culture towards obesity by being proactive not reactive.

What I do mean is that we can a proverbial protractor to draw the contrast line between from my advisor's zealous proactive actions to our apathetic reactive environment.

He's not even 100% certain that all the information in that textbook will ever be applicable. Yet the *chance* that this may *one day* be useful is more than enough to motivate him.

We can only hope to be such a galvanized fulcrum of psychological practices to impact the systems around us utilizing all available emotional resources. As we've seen in the previous chapter the current and future circumstances are dire.

These five methods of self-improvement range from the moderately established (Counseling) to the relatively unrenowned (Affirmations) within our USA culture.

Again, the cultural shift we're chasing isn't just about these five practices, it's about being proactive and not reactive towards our emotions and ultimately, to our fitness.

1. **Counseling.**
2. **Sleep Training.**
3. **Meditations.**
4. **Mindfulness.**
5. **Affirmations.**

As we've seen in the previous chapter, many of the economic effects of obesity are being felt in the international community. However, for our greater American society, much of these five methods are outside of our collective comfort zones. To our American eyes and ears, they can appear and sound: hokey, lacking credibility, and overly sentimental.

These five can conjure comparisons to tarot cards and mystic psychics staring into crystal balls with a large head-wrap. Critics of many of these methods have been specific in their rebuttal and will be addressed within this same chapter.

I assert that as discussed in previous chapters, we're not in this solely for personal growth. These five methods are not limited to an EQ-enhanced journey towards improved fitness. This entire section of chapters 11-15 is about Impacting the systems that can become obstacles on that journey.

My advisor left no proverbial stone unturned. Our goal is just as robust: A healthier, happier, more economically sound America that won't have to decide one day between funding our local elementary schools versus treating our obese population at the local hospital. If *one* person drops 10% body fat percentage points or becomes more self-forgiving while being biometrically fit because they got a favorable "Tarot Card Reading" then all of us need to be happier because our country's economic weight of treating obesity is one person lighter.

1. Counseling

Go back to Tom from the gym. He can discuss with his counselor and reflect later as to why his subconscious is protecting him from "embarrassment" lifting next to the guy pushing 315 pounds. He can also discuss why he feels, or more accurately, *fears* everyone in the gym is paying attention to him in the first place.

Tom is symptomatic of our American culture where self-reliance and "toughness" are highly valued. Therefore, seeking counseling might be seen as a weakness, contradicting these values.

Tom impacts our system by not being of the 11% of Americans with a gym membership that visits once a month or less. If we can't coalesce to get my colleagues/friends who collectively embody "Tom" to seek counseling, then the price to pay is the increased economic spiral from chapter 13.

The good news. Of these five, counseling is becoming more accepted in our general society. Barriers do exist in the form of insurance coverage, finances, and time-availability of quality counselors.

2. Sleep training:

We talked about obstacles like procrastination and fear as early as chapter 1. Sleep training is about creating new habits.

We can literally ask our subconscious for answers as we sleep. There are a thunderous number of articles and blogs on the subject (even a quote from Thomas Edison) so I'll summarize:

- When everything else is off (devices and televisions). Clothes and work items put away and done. The only thing left for you to do is fall asleep. You're in bed, head on the pillow.
- Think about your problem/question.
- Hold the question/problem in your head for as long as possible. SAM will work on it while you sleep. It doesn't sleep. You do.
- *Visualize* your goals being met. In as much detail as possible.
- Go to sleep looking forward to more clarity when you awaken.

There are numerous applications for this type of self-help. I can't help but think of our stripper from Chapter 7. She only has one problem or question to ask/solve before dosing off: "How can I be better at planning my day"?

3. Meditation

Even though meditation has been around for 5000 years, it has barely been on *this* continent for 100 years. And to be honest, I didn't know what to think of it as an avenue to help with fitness.

In fact, I barely knew anything about it overall. I heard it was a good way to relax and or focus.

The only things I knew about how to "relax" was to:

- Have a drink?
- Maybe get a massage?
- Take a nap?
- All three in that order?

There are just as many varieties of meditations as there are companies that make high blood pressure medications.

- Breath-related meditations.
- Mantra-based.
- Guided.
- Visualization.

But what are the benefits of meditation in terms of physical health?

- Reduces Stress/Anxiety. This can help directly with our Fat-Shaming stress society increasing biomarkers in our diagnostics.
- Helps Sleep and Memory.
- Increases Self-Awareness.

While the first two are great, the third item is the jackpot for our purposes. This is exactly what we're trying to figure out: ourselves. What is our emotional attachment to things that are in our way of our physical health? How can we envision our journey towards better fitness as fun and enjoyable, not a lengthy stay in a prison?

Just like the gym, which is just a place where we attempt to be in better physical condition by repeatedly exercising our skeletal muscles and our heart; Meditation is a place where we attempt to be in better emotional condition by repeatedly exercising our ability to learn about ourselves.

Both the gym and meditation can help us look and feel stronger about our individual selves.

Application: My friend who wants to lose weight is not healthy biometrically. However, her stress level from not being comfortable with her weight is just as much an issue.

4. Mindfulness

"Mindfulness is the simple act of paying attention and noticing and being present in whatever you're doing. When you are being actively mindful, you are noticing the world around you, as well as your thoughts, feelings and behaviors, movement and affects you have on others around you." (Zeidman, 2022)

Mindfulness can be part of meditation. It helps with our focus.

Focus. Let's get a show of hands on how many of us are juggling, work, family, errands, plus a hobby that we hope develop into a side-money-making plan? And trying to lose weight must fit inside our whole frantic lives.

Our thoughts can race ahead towards thinking about the future of all these things we're juggling. Simple thoughts about what will happen a month away, or 12 months away in life, especially when we have desires to be in better shape and in a better place financially as well.

In the next 30 seconds, with our racing minds, we think about what we could have done better in the situations that led up to this moment. Or we think about:

- Bad past relationships that contributed to our current situation.
- Jobs that didn't and still don't pay enough money.
- The errands and tasks we need to run this weekend. Upcoming social events.

We don't have the mental space to even focus on fitness at this moment, so let's put it off until Monday.

Focusing the mind on a particular object, thought, or activity – to train attention and self-awareness. That's sounds great but what we really want is the mental clarity and emotional calmness to not just tackle our issues, but not being stressed while doing it.

Curiosity and Anxiety about the future in addition to frustrations about the past can rob us all from our attention to the only thing we can control: This moment right now!

We're talking about being present because remember, SAM doesn't understand "past" or "future". It doesn't comprehend that you want to be in better financial or physical shape 12 months from now.

Be present for your present.

The direct application for a character from our book: That would be the author who is dazzled by the bar scenes in big cities, small towns, and cruise ships. Mindfulness has absolutely gotten my racing brain to slow down enough to push back from the bar scene and focus. If you're reading this, then these words in this paragraph are the payoff.

5. Affirmations

One of the goals of being a trainer or a Pilates instructor wasn't just to guide individuals through a physical workout, it was to encourage them to believe they could accomplish their goal.

Sometimes the encouragement was just to finish a particular exercise. But at the end of the workout, it's to encourage them to continue along this path towards fitness, even when we're not physically together. A pep-talk.

"Generally speaking, affirmations are used to reprogram the subconscious mind, to encourage us to believe certain things about ourselves or about the world and our place within it. They are also used to help us create the reality we want." (Lively, 2014)

Affirmations are literally taking time out to speak directly to SAM to encourage it towards goals you would like. A pep-talk.

Speak to it in the present tense. SAM doesn't understand last week or next month. And make it reality based. (And yes, use the word "I". You can't literally address your subconscious as "SAM" it's just a metaphor.)

The proper way to use affirmations is not: *"I am a CEO"* or *"I am in great shape now"*. Those might be your goals. But those are not reality, and your subconscious will call: *"Nonsense"*.

Instead say:

- "I am strategizing on how to become a CEO and I enjoy the process."
- "I enjoy working on all aspects of my fitness journey and I'm happy."

It's a simple statement. You take time to speak it to yourself to encourage and enhance your emotional disposition.

And just like exercise, you'll get better at it overtime. You can't lose 10 or 50 or 100 pounds in one day, you work on it.

Critics abound

The Skeptical Inquirer magazine criticized the lack of falsifiability and testability of these claims (meditations, affirmations). Physicist Ali Alousi, for instance, criticized it as unmeasurable and questioned the likelihood that thoughts can affect anything outside of the head. In addition, critics have asserted that the evidence provided is usually anecdotal and that, because of the self-selecting disposition of the positive feedback, as well as the selective nature of any results, these reports are susceptible to confirmation bias and selection bias. (Alousi, 2007)

Oh great. A physicist says this is all *"nonsense"*.

I'd love to sit down with him and ask:

> "What about the emotional manipulation of the food, restaurant, or entertainment industries? Are those unmeasurable?

Do their actions affect anything on their revenues or our waistlines?

Again, to be clear: Our western culture is not quite adroit at accepting these five practices as commonplace. In that sense, Ali Alousi is mostly correct.

Emotional Wellness is not measurable by our western standards. We can't graph it. We can't project or extrapolate any of it into the future metric-defined quandary to create a future meeting in Mississippi. Our society (I'm entirely guilty of this mind-set) wants facts, figures, and tangible ideologies that we can put on a spreadsheet or PowerPoint presentation slides. We want our culture to continue to be corporate.

Stockholders want quantifiable data to review, not nebulous concepts. That's our culture, like it or not. We'll get to stockholders and capitalism directly next chapter, but first:

I would counter to critics of these five methods, that our subconscious minds are already on spreadsheets and board-room presentations. Check the industries we've named and put the indirectly stress-inducing medical community and life science industries on that list as well.

Put the revenues from those industries in one column. Compare that to the expenses of state & commercial insurances spent on obesity related illnesses in another column. You can make all the graphs and charts you want from there.

(I would do it myself, but while the food, restaurant, Hollywood, social media, and pharmaceutical companies all make their revenues known as individual stock-tradeable companies, I would need to clone myself several times to research and compile those figures into in one document. Plus, I currently view *accounting* as a jail sentence.)

We're capable of being just like my former advisor: Using our intellectual capacity to our advantage. We just need the motivation to be proactive and the temerity to change our culture.

The statistics from Chapter 13 have already been trending in one direction for decades and nothing has altered their trajectory to this point.

Solving this cultural conundrum is going to be challenging. Individual emotional intelligence to increase collective fitness will need a boost from many different participants. Those participants need to be influential enough to focus our societal lens on fitness. And they need an incentive.

Thanks to the folks in Athens. We'll head back up north. I can do some of my best thinking in the car. On the open road. Let's get back on the highway.

CHAPTER 15

Conclusions

THE ROAD TO CHANGE

Back on the highway. No music, no phone calls.

Just thoughts.

That conference in Philly was lacking one thing: An ability to reach the emotions of the people that were not present.

It was such a helpful event for patients with that rare genetic lung disease who were present. But data and experts weren't enough to reach the thousands of individuals who may carry the genes but emotionally elected not to attend.

Transitioning, we mentioned in chapter 7 that individual habits and beliefs take time to change. But we're out of time according to the sobering statistics and trends from chapter 13. We can't alter the trajectory of those trends merely with experts narrating PowerPoint slides at a conference. Not because those presentations aren't worthy, but we're preaching to the proverbial choir.

The ramifications of our lack of emotional self-awareness and self-regulation manifest in our fitness and obesity trends, mainly due to the rise of manipulative marketing that originates in the 1970s and 80s.

Those entities aren't going to stop. Food Manufacturing, entertainment, restaurants, even the corporate conglomerates that reside over our healthcare and insurance industries – not one of them are going to alter their long-range business plans to the point our fitness and obesity trends decelerate.

Those industries fully captivate our subconscious. From dim lights at pricey restaurants to social media algorithms designed to fixate on an app for hours. Bemoaning those systems' current manipulations is catalytically wasted energy – and we need all the energy we can generate for this endeavor.

We're also continuing the trends of throwing money at diet fads and gyms, spinning the hamster wheel of fitness. Our biomarkers – whether from fat-shaming stress or fatness alone will continue to send us to the hospitals, burning a hole in our state and national budgets.

Capitalism

We've taken a lot of direct and indirect shots at the economic system of capitalism. I personally think capitalism leads to irreproachable innovation and that innovation produces an ever-increasing quality number of products and services. Capitalism breeds competition and leads to a form of self-regulation: Either you make a product or service that citizens need, or they will spend their money elsewhere.

But capitalism can also be self-serving inside of one company or one industry. I wish we were in a different human evolutionary phase where our collective monetary myopic nature wasn't restricting us from reaching our fitness aspirations. However, we can create incentives for existing companies to be more efficient toward their own capitalistic endpoints. We just need to show one industry that there is unrealized potential effectiveness for their existing systems.

I mentioned in the previous chapter that being proactive not reactive and being willing to do "whatever it takes" is needed for us to solve our current and future obesity trends. Well, that's only as good of a sentiment as we can culturally integrate it into our capitalistic society. I wish we could produce a list of non-profit organizations who prioritize obesity and/or promote fitness. However, none of them have the financial teeth or societal reach to battle the mammoth industries that manipulate SAM.

The solution to that equation from chapter 1 will take a classic multi-pronged approach from various organizations and industries. Some of these entities are not engaged in making a capitalistic profit. I'm bringing up capitalism as a sub chapter not to compare it to other economic systems, but to show that not all these entities that can help us are in it for the money.

The collaboration of these entities is The REDI Network.

Some units within this network will help to the full limit of their capacity. Their ideologies are a perfect match for this endeavor even if their societal reach is limited.

But as we'll see, there is one entity that is financially incentivized and culturally influential enough to be the full bearer of this weighty task.

The six entities of the REDI Network:

1. Pharmaceutical Assistance Programs.

My conscious emotions. On that original drive from Philly, I really thought this entity could be the single missing variable for the whole equation. I thought of how much directly assisting the fitness/obesity crises could enhance this industry's collective corporate brands. I thought about their tremendous reach into our communities at the doctor's office, the hospital, your local pharmacy, and direct-to-consumer advertising.

I thought these programs would be perfect. The goals of these programs are to assist people in getting medicine at little or no cost when individuals don't have the finances or insurance to afford/cover it. All I need to do is make sure all medications treating obesity related illness now factor in a component to track the fitness/BMI of the patients.

I've promoted these programs – with their shiny, laminated brochures - directly to Dr. Smith in her office and I've educated her staff on how "we" (my employer) can help.

Hard truth: I never heard any success stories from the doc or the staff on how these programs helped *one* patient. I know the office staff tried and I'm sure it happened. I'm sure there are patients out there who couldn't afford XYZ medication, called up the hotline and with help from the office staff and it all worked out.

In reality. The coverage gaps between insurance, financial eligibility, and formulary status are notoriously confusing to patients and providers. To be honest, even as a former employee (who hates conspiracy theories) I can't help but wonder if the eligibility status criteria is deliberately vague.

And although Pharma companies - like Novo Nordisk - are currently funding a lot of well-rounded obesity research, pharmaceutical companies making meds related to obesity-related illnesses are also gaining in this excess spending we outlined in chapter 13.

Costs for you equals revenue for me. Those rising healthcare costs are going towards our hospital health care systems (coming up next) and the medications we consume. Therefore, it would be ethically responsible, yet economically not incentivized for these two industries to change the culture of the American Obesity epidemic.

Their incentive to collaborate on this journey is still my original thought: Increasing their corporate brand footprint. Cardiology, Endocrinology, even Rheumatology medical brands can benefit from being associated with other corporate entities who are in the fight against obesity.

2. Hospital Health Systems.

This is not merely referring to your neighborhood hospital.

I walked through a ton of local and regional hospitals speaking with doctors and administrators in the beginning of my career. The last few years, barely any of them are still independent entities. Just today, *two* more local hospitals have been purchased by conglomerate organizations in the time it took you to read this paragraph. Maybe three.

They have been acquired to create mega hospital systems, which now dominate the economics of our healthcare facilities. Those systems have tens of thousands of employees doing rounds, working with the exact patients where obesity-related illness is manifested. For our purposes in fitness/obesity, this leads to one huge problem.

While the doctors, nurses, and staff all individually strive to make positive changes in their patients' lives, all the additional "costs" we saw escalating in Chapter 13 are converted to *revenue* for these conglomerates (just like pharma).

Example. HCA Healthcare, the nation's largest health system as of January 2024, has "41,000+ beds in 219 hospitals and a net-patient revenue of $49.2M". (DefintiveHealthcare, 2024).

Add in other conglomerates like Trinity, Kaiser, Ascension, and you have business entities that are *not* directly emotionally manipulating our subconscious (leading to our fitness/obesity crises) but are reaping the financial benefits, nonetheless.

What incentive could the business personnel (not the medical employees) possibly have towards decelerating those trends we've outlined? Yes, obesity rates are reaching dangerous levels. Yes, their own employees are overworked and at the limits (especially the pathologists and lab personnel at these local and regional hospitals who can't outsource their pathology needs fast enough to companies like LabCorp with the recently acquired BioReference and Quest subsidiaries like AmeriPath).

Hard truth: There aren't many financial incentives for large groups to examine current obesity trends and subsequently sprint to assist. These entities do have incredible capabilities of reaching people in key problem areas: Low-income urban and remote/rural communities. In fact, that reach can be exactly the problem.

"A large health system that acquires a small rural hospital may be less responsive to community needs and more willing to eliminate service lines, such as obstetric care. Relatedly, a hospital may also reduce spending on community benefits after being acquired by a health system." (Godwin, 2023)

Still. They are the first line of defense. I would urge the medical employees of these entities to engage with their counterparts in the Obesity non-profits (coming up next) to pressure – and that's the right word – the parent companies to alert patients of the wellness programs offered by commercial and state insurances. Especially in the smaller hospitals in rural and urban areas.

3. Obesity non-profits.

- The Obesity Society. A scientific membership organization. An expert-level assortment of physicians and scientific researchers.
- Obesity Action Coalition. 80,000 members strong, it exists for those affected by obesity.
- American Obesity Foundation. Focuses on obesity-related diseases.

These are full of people who genuinely care about this issue and fully realize the social and health ramifications of fitness. These organizations remind me directly of that conference in Philadelphia: Awesome people but lacking a footprint large enough to reach individuals who aren't already directly affiliated. Sadly, for all of us, not enough people have heard of them.

Their function in this equation is specific. They are keenly aware of the disease-states and cascading effects of obesity, so working with the hospital conglomerates from a corporate level (with their regulating medical boards) to pinpoint how to chart and track progress.

They are a full-fledged consultant for this endeavor. They're already a proactive, culturally integrated, research-based entity and perfect for this journey.

4. National Academy of Sports Medicine (NASM) and other personal trainer/fitness organizations.

The gyms in our country absolutely have the cultural weight, but we're already getting people *into* the gyms and studios, we're not getting enough to stay engaged to reach their fitness goals. Tom is still being intimidated daily across the country. Conversely, the stripper's emotional connections to her lifestyle will still overshadow her fitness goals. Both walked through the doors of the gym on their own and neither reached their goals.

Personal trainers, fitness coaches - and dieticians – with a little bit of training on EQ, can make a huge difference. The limiting factor is still, we're not reaching people who aren't going to the gym. Trainers – with or without EQ training - are only accessible for people who physically walk through those doors. Just like the conference in Philly, we're not reaching people who aren't there.

But I can grip this steering wheel tightly on this drive thinking about how many trainers like me could benefit from even the slightest bit of EQ knowledge. I could speak to my friends and family who collectively personify "Tom" and I could see better results from all clients who struggled with their emotional attachment to their current lifestyle.

5. EQ Foundations

- International Society for Emotional Intelligence. Now we're talking. They utilize scientific approaches towards solving issues in business and medicine (and others). They provide research and collaborative information for governments and organizations. Awesome. Limiting reagent: if you've never heard of EQ, you're not seeking them out. Covalent bond potential: They are culturally focused on collaboration and increasing individual and social well-being.

- Consortium for Emotional Intelligence Organizations. This is the EQ version of the Peter G. Peterson Foundation: A research think-tank. While they're mostly focusing on workplace applications of emotional intelligence, getting their experts on board with a national crisis as big as obesity would be critical. More specifically, we need them to work directly with our mitochondrial engine in this journey – the one industry that makes this ride possible.

- Six Seconds. The international Emotional Intelligence Network. The EQ international version of NASM: Certifying thousands of individuals to coach others in emotional intelligence. And that's exactly where we need them, and organizations like them to pitch in: Training the personal trainers and dieticians of whom fitness-seeking citizens are already seeking (after they get back from their cruises).

These foundations can assist every single other entity within this network. They specifically work with NASM through the Wellness programs coming up next.

6. Insurance Wellness and Fitness Programs.

Funded. Incentivized. Culturally integrated. Striving to be proactive. The currently existing Wellness Programs of top insurance companies can coordinate all the entities along this journey.

One of their best attributes is their reach. They have access to more people - obese, overweight, fit – than these other entities. Not everyone visits the hospital. Not everyone needs pharmaceutical meds. But most of us have either commercial or government health insurance.

"In 2021, private health insurance coverage continued to be more prevalent than public coverage, at 66.0 percent and 35.7 percent, respectively. Of the subtypes of health insurance coverage, employer-based insurance was the most common, covering 54.3 percent of the population for some or all of the calendar year, followed by Medicaid (18.9 percent), Medicare (18.4 percent), and direct-purchase coverage (10.2 percent)." (Keisler-Starkey, 2022)

Their reach is good; however, they still have limitations which we'll get to momentarily. Wellness programs' number one contribution to this journey is that they are already in these spaces.

There are existing programs for gyms, alcohol abuse, quitting smoking and yes, obesity issues. In addition, some programs such as Anthem's Employee Assistance Programs work with behavioral health experts to improve emotional stress levels.

Therein lies opportunity number one. An unaccounted variable in this fitness/obesity equation is the psychological link connecting subconscious emotions to physical fitness. Yes, some of them treat emotional stress as well as physical fitness. Not all of them treat the whole person. From Chapter 1:

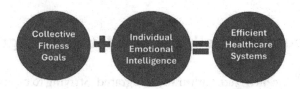

These programs need to fully retire the concept of putting their sub-programs into silos if they want to increase their effectiveness. By all accounts, the effectiveness, i.e. the Return-On-Investment of these costly programs has been substandard. The following quote shows we're only capturing part of the workforce – and not the ones we want in order to change our obesity metrics.

(Wellness Programs have) "mixed data on program effectiveness. Early reports on WHPs oversold their effectiveness, with more rigorous studies indicating that most WHP initiatives typically engage individuals who are already pursuing healthy lifestyles." (Weinsten, 2022)

To be clear, some of them are doing just that and even adding financial assistance to employees as well.

"Leaders now recognize well-being as a holistic, multi-dimensional phenomenon. Because well-being is complex and multi-faceted, there is ample room for individuals to differ in their wellness needs. For example, some may have their physical health in order but struggle with their financial wellness. Others may be thriving financially while suffering emotionally. As a result, programs that contain offerings to help employees achieve or maintain wellness in every domain are much more likely to garner high participation rates." (Wellable, 2024)

What was that final phrase? Participation rates.

Despite the evolution of these programs to cater to the whole person and despite their reach into most of the societal spaces we need them to be, the single damming reason that Insurance Wellness programs aren't seeing the results they want is:

An employee like me.

I've gone into detail to lead off chapters in this book with anecdotes from my time in various corporate jobs and it's impossible to believe: None of these huge Pharma, Lab Diagnostic, or Scientific Laboratory Supply companies ever saw one second of participation from me in their Insurance Wellness Programs.

For two decades.

Why?

I never heard of them.

Ever.

"If wellness programs are in high demand, why are 75% of the employees who have access to them not participating?" (Wellable, 2024)

I had to go back to the websites of the insurance companies that covered me in my time as an employee in these high-profile companies. I checked to make sure they even had these programs while I was in Vegas, or under the tent at NIH or... driving home from that conference I just left to climb into this company car. They did: Aetna Wellness, Humana Go365, BCBS CareFirst Well-Being.

Ironically, I'm in their target group: Workout enthusiasts.

To that point about target groups, and continuing about participation rates, these programs have traditionally struggled to get participation from the employees that need their services the most – our obese/overweight population - the folks at the buffet from the cruise. A lot of them don't think they can succeed in the fitness universe, so they don't try (people just want to stay in their comfort zones). Another component of *this* group is that they don't want the company to know about their health (privacy concerns are real in healthcare, of course).

But if these programs are missing me, they're missing other folks who could benefit - but don't know they exist. There are other employees who know they *exist* but not really to what extent.

I am more "flabber-and-ghasted" to find out in my research for this book that there were *financial incentives* for me to stay in shape via wellness programs at my job than I was to find out restaurants and bars are manipulating my subconscious via lights, music, and chairs. These companies need just as much noise around their wellness programs as that Pharma Vegas opening event. You can't have employees start any job in the training stage without realizing the wellness opportunities available to them. Employee, meet Wellness Program. Wellness Program, meet our new employee, Jay Houston.

But we never got introduced.

Make no mistake, while I was a personal trainer and a Pilates instructor and a youth football coach - all fitness-based activities – I was still employed full time day-by-day, week-by-week by those companies with these programs. The metrics that they use to track fitness and retain me as a healthy, happy employee would have been something I would have strived to achieve.

Here I am, driving in this car trying to brainstorm about a network of entities capable of EQ-foundation coaches who coordinate with personal trainers with an extension to research-based obesity societies and my former pharmaceutical PAPs. And while I'm churning that around in my head, I'm not aware whatsoever of the current wellness entity available to me. I have the insurance card right in my wallet in my pocket, it's with me on this drive. But I had no idea.

Extrapolating: it's not merely the "fear of having to change" like that lady said at that meeting I just left. A large part of those Staggering Resources met with Thunderous Apathy derives from not knowing an organization for patients with a rare genetic lung disease existed in the first place.

Changing the culture of the country means finding ways to alert its citizens that there are options to do so.

The solution. Coordinate entities into a network. Show the Wellness programs how to reach: me. Because they didn't, despite me religiously checking my company emails for *all* things work-related.

Doing my due diligence before sitting down to type all of this. I spoke directly to people who work in this field (wellness insurance) who are trying daily to connect employees to their wellness programs. I found one common issue: Mid and upper-level managers within the company. Not the insurance companies. My employers

Many of the managers I've worked for directly and overlapped with their sales/consulting territories are only vaguely aware of these programs and more importantly, don't see the benefits to their direct employee reports.

Bluntly, upon further reflection, many mid-level managers that I've worked with directly lack self-awareness as part of EQ. Their focus is consciously on increased sales numbers or increased influence with disease-state-thought-leaders to facilitate themselves moving up the corporate ladder. Those subconscious motivations to move up the corporate ladder are frequently to compensate for real or perceived slights in their upbringing.

Hence, they wouldn't concern themselves about helping the wellness of their employees because they would be troubled by the idea of their direct reports (me) taking their eyes off the proverbial ball. Managers with a subconscious desire for external validation want employees 100% focused on increasing sales/influence as a function of helping them climb the ladder through outlined company metrics.

It's the same fear of leaving a comfort zone that the relatives of that genetic lung disorder feel when presented with the opportunity for that cheek swab.

Fair balance: It's not all managers. However, some of the mid-level managers who do possess EQ can become burned out dealing with the constant non-EQ managers around them and especially above them on the workforce ladder.

The core issue is this. Far too many managers with influence within the organization are there to be validated by their title and the success they bring to their company through metrics. *If they knew* they could get better metrics by implementing EQ tactics for their employees through wellness programs, they *might* try it. But it would have to start with their own self-reflection. Their own vulnerability. And that's a difficult highway to maneuver.

But we have no choice. The data from Chapter 13 is not going to get better by coddling the subconscious motivations of mid-to upper-level managers who could disperse information to their direct reports. Who gets this started?

This author, as well as others on this journey.

As an individual who has worked in many aspects of these industries compiled in this book yet was not "found" by employee wellness programs.

Going forward, focusing on company employees with commercial (in the future, government) insurance can assist local, regional, and national statistics and gives us all a tangible target: The flattening of those surging obesity trends from Chapter 13.

These wellness programs need the entities from previous pages of this chapter for maximum efficiency. A separate line of coaches trained in EQ foundation principles to coordinate with personal trainers from various gym organizations. Part of EQ training is dealing with the fear some employees have of their information getting back to the company – we'll all be here to help - not leak data. And by alert, I mean directly speak to the subtle, subconscious manipulations by various industries and how to absorb it with EQ to reach all personal goals.

Wellness programs must incorporate data directly from the Obesity foundations and our friends at NIH Obesity research task force on the delicate topics of Fat Shaming and Body Positivity and the effects on biomarkers.

Personal trainers like the 2009 version of me, with even the *minimal* amount of EQ training would know how to address the obstacle of my clients' emotional attachments to their lifestyles. I could speak even minimally on how to be more vulnerable and utilize accessible counseling, meditation-training, and mindfulness from coordinated wellness programs would maximize Tom pushing through his fears and pushing up his bench press. EQ coaches can have employees less intimidated by the vast information discussed in chapter 11. We'll all have the "whatever-it-takes" demeanor from chapter 14.

As currently existing, here is a limiting reagent: Available counselors. Those EQ trained coaches available for one-on-one work with an employee aren't sitting on shelves like meds in a drug closet. We'll need to train more via the EQ foundations that certify people in that arena.

All coordinated entities help the overall lack of efficacy which currently exists. Despite the investments made by insurance companies, numerous articles suggest that wellness programs have had only minor impacts on health markers. They are helping with weight management and exercise, but they have not significantly affected clinical health, healthcare spending, absenteeism, or job performance.

Best yet, unlike Hospitals systems or Pharma who would have to see less patients in their facilities and less prescription, insurances companies wouldn't have to lose any existing revenue while improving their own societal footprint. Insurance companies will still draw revenue from covering all of us. So again, here's the final version of that equation from Chapter 1:

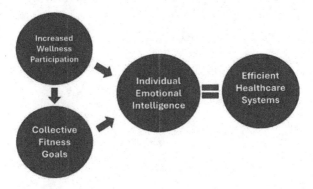

Deep breath... I can daydream while I'm still in this car... back to one of those bars on that cruise. None of this was churning around in my brain. It was so sunny. It was so relaxing.

Do you think if we build a network and show companies how to steer more people into wellness and we subsequently slow down obesity trends by linking EQ to fitness... do you think insurance companies will lower the premiums that they charge employers and put more money back in our pockets?

(Looks both ways. Sips drink.)

Another question for you while we're at this sun-filled bar on this ship:

Do you think EQ can help us with the delicate topics of Politics and Media?

We won't get into it now, but man oh man do I have a personal Narcissism saga to share with you. It ties into Donald Trump, of all people.

We'll save that for another time. Let's get another round.

Special Thanks

Ann Houston
Leah Tanou
Dr. Stephanie Evans-Byrd
Dr. Curtis Byrd
Bikram Yoga Works

BIBLIOGRAPHY

Agency, C. I. (2017). *The World Factbook.*

Alousi, A. (2007, April). *Skeptical Inquirer.*

Baracz, S. (2018, August 30). *Pudmed.* Retrieved from NCCBI: https://pubmed.ncbi.nlm.nih.gov/30172802/

Beiner, A. (2017, March 7). *National Center for Biotech Info.* Retrieved from PubMed: https://www.ncbi.nlm.nih.gov/pmc/articles/ PMC5359159/

Belluz, J. (2023, March 15). *STAT.* Retrieved from Report: Obesity could cost the world over $4 trillion a year by 2035: https://www. statnews.com/2023/03/02/obesity-costs-4-trillion-2035/

Block, R. D. (n.d.). Former President, American Academy of Pediatrics.

Cawley, J. (2021, January 20). *JMCP.* Retrieved from Direct medical costs of obesity in the United States and the most populous states: https://www.jmcp.org/doi/full/10.18553/jmcp.2021.20410

Chan, T. (2024). *Harvard School of Public Health.* Retrieved from https://www.hsph.harvard.edu/obesity-prevention-source/ obesity-consequences/economic/#references

Clear, J. (n.d.). Retrieved from JamesClear.com

CornellUniversity. (2018, Feb 8). Science Daily. p. https://www. sciencedaily.com/releases/2018/02/180208180356.htm.

Daley, B. (2017, August 9). *TheConversation.com.*

DualDiagnosis.org, F. R. (n.d.).

Duckworth, A. (n.d.). *angeladuckworth.com.*

Goswami,J.H.(2012,March). *Well.org.*RetrievedfromAspireInfinitus: https://well.org/mindset/how-your-subconscious-mind-controls-your-behavior/

Gough, C. (2017). US Health Clubs and Fitness Centers. In *US Health Clubs and Fitness Centers.*

Harfman, B. (2021, December 27). *Beverage Industry.* Retrieved from Beverage Industry.com: https://www.bevindustry.com/ articles/94682-weight-management-coincides-with-healthier-lifestyle#:~:text=An%20estimated%2045%20million%20 Americans%20go%20on%20a,health%20issues%20like%20 heart%20disease%2C%20diabetes%20and%20hypertension.

Harrington, J. (2023, March 13). *Tempo.* Retrieved from 24/7Tempo: https://247tempo.com/states-with-the-highest-diabetes-rates/?utm_ source=msn&utm_medium=referral&utm_campaign=msn&utm_ content=states-with-the-highest-diabetes-rates&wsrlui=47228021

Li, e. a. (2020). C-Reactive Protein Causes Adult-Onset Obesity Through Chronic Inflammatory Mechanism. *Frontiers in Cell and Developmental Biology,* https://www.ncbi.nlm.nih.gov/pmc/articles/ PMC7044181/#:~:text=As%20a%20signature%20marker%20 for%20systemic%20inflammations%2C%20C-reactive,by%20a%20 statistical%20approach%20%28Timpson%20et%20al.%2C%20 2011%29.

Lipton, B. (n.d.). *BruceLipton.com*. Retrieved from brucelipton.com

Lively, K. (2014, March 12). *Smart Relationships*. Retrieved from Psychology Today: https://www.psychologytoday.com/us/ blog/smart-relationships/201403/affirmations-the-why-what-how-and-what-if

Lopez, C. (2020). *Milken Institute*. Retrieved from Weighing Down America: https://milkeninstitute.org/sites/default/files/reports-pdf/Weighing%20Down%20America%20v12.3.20_0.pdf

Manson, M. (n.d.). *MarkManson.net*. Retrieved from MarkManson.net

McDermott, J. (2019, April). *Finder.com*. Retrieved from Huffington Post, USA Today.

Nam, G. (2021, June 23). *NIh.gov*. Retrieved from NIH.gov: https:// www.ncbi.nlm.nih.gov/pmc/articles/PMC8277583/

Nuccio, S. (2012). *https://www.sylvianenuccio.com/*. Retrieved from Subconscious Mind: https://www.sylvianenuccio.com/

Peterson. (n.d.). *https://www.pgpf.org/finding-solutions/healthcare*. Retrieved from https://www.pgpf.org/finding-solutions/ healthcare: https://www.pgpf.org/finding-solutions/healthcare

Puiu, T. (2020, February 11). ZMEScience.com.

Richardson. (1961). Cultural uniformity in reaction to physical disabilities. *American Sociology Review*.

Rubin, G. (n.d.). *inc.com*. Retrieved from Why you shouldn't reward yourself for good habits: inc.com

Signs.com. (2014). Retrieved from Blog 2014: Signs.com

Sirota, M. M. (n.d.). *Huffington Post*.

Thompson, D. (2024, Jan 16). Higher Premiums for Employer-Sponsored Insurance Keep Wages Low: Study. *US News and World Report*, pp. https://www.usnews.com/news/health-news/articles/2024-01-16/higher-premiums-for-employer-sponsored-insurance-keep-wages-low-study.

Tomiyama. (2018, August). *NIH*. Retrieved from NIH Biotechnology Centers for Info: https://pubmed.ncbi.nlm.nih.gov/30107800/

USAFacts.org. (2020, Feb 1). Obesity rates nearly tripled over the last 50 years.

Wang, C. (2015, November). Health Affairs. *Severe Obesity In Adults Cost State Medicaid Programs Nearly $8 Billion In 2013*, p. https://www.healthaffairs.org/doi/10.1377/hlthaff.2015.0633.

Ward, Z. (2021, March 24). *PLOS One*. Retrieved from Association of bodymassindexwithhealthcareexpendituresintheUnitedStatesby ageandsex: https://journals.plos.org/plosone/article?id=10.1371/journal.pone.0247307

Werle, C. (2014, May). *Springer.com*. Retrieved from Is it fun or is it excercise: Springer.com

Williams, J. (2020, Feb 3). *US News and World Report*. Retrieved from https://www.usnews.com/news/healthiest-communities/articles/2020-02-03/body-positivity-weight-bias-and-the-battle-for-a-healthy-life

WorldObesity.org. (2023). *WorldObesity.org*. Retrieved from https://www.worldobesityday.org/resources/entry/world-obesity-atlas-2023

Yashi, K. (2023, June 19). Obesity and type 2 diabetes. *StatPearls*, pp. https://www.ncbi.nlm.nih.gov/books/NBK592412/#:~:text=The%20lifetime%20diabetes%20risk%20in%20men%20older%20than, diabetes%20is%20indicated%20in%20all%20patients%20with%20obesity.

Zeidman, E. (2022, May 11). *The Benefits of Mindfulness Meditation for Cognitive Health and Learning*. Retrieved from chopra.com: https://chopra.com/blogs/meditation/the-benefits-of-mindfulness-meditation-for-cognitive-health-and-learning

Printed in the United States
by Baker & Taylor Publisher Services

Printed in the United States
by Baker & Taylor Publisher Services